STAYING HEALTHY

Nutrition, Lifestyle & Medicine

Timely Reports to Keep
Journalists, Scholars and the Public
Abreast of Developing Issues, Events and Trends

Editorial Research Reports
Published by Congressional Quarterly Inc.
1414 22nd Street, N.W.
Washington, D.C. 20037

About the Cover

The cover was designed by Staff Artist Belle Burkhart.

Editor, Hoyt Gimlin
Managing Editor, Sandra Stencel
Editorial Assistants, Laurie De Maris, Elizabeth Furbush
Production Manager, I. D. Fuller
Assistant Production Manager, Maceo Mayo

Library of Congress Cataloging in Publication Data

Main entry under title:

Editorial research reports on staying healthy.

Bibliography: p.
Includes index.
1. Health — Addresses, essays, lectures. 2. Nutrition — Addresses, essays, lectures. 3. Medicine — Addresses, essays, lectures.
   I. Educational research reports. II. Congressional Quarterly, inc.

RA776.5.E34   1984   613   83-15292
ISBN 0-87187-278-1

Contents

Foreword

Americans spent over $320 billion on health care in 1982 — an amount equal to 10 percent of the nation's gross national product. Rising health care costs are one reason for the growing interest in preventive medicine. Increasing numbers of people are trying to improve their health by changing their lifestyles and eating habits. They're exercising more and consuming less tobacco, alcohol, salt, sugar, fat and caffeine.

In their efforts to stay healthy, Americans are getting a lot of support from their employers, who have discovered that it is cheaper to keep workers healthy than to pay for their illnesses. In recent years, thousands of companies have set up some type of physical fitness program for employees. Often these include not only exercise facilities, but also programs on nutrition, smoking, weight-control, stress management, alcohol and drug abuse, and similar topics.

The benefits of preventive medicine are also recognized by physicians and other health professionals. Doctors frequently "prescribe" regular exercise as a way to increase overall health and reduce the risk of developing a number of serious health problems, especially cardiovascular disease. More than 2,500 hospitals now offer some type of health-promotion program, according to the American Hospital Association. Some 400 hospitals have constructed fitness facilities within the hospital grounds.

Meanwhile, medical research has produced new discoveries in the treatment and cure of cancer, in the importance of sleeping and dreaming, and in the alleviation of chronic pain. Doctors are also reassessing the care and treatment of the nation's mentally ill.

The ten Reports that make up this book examine all these issues in detail, providing a clear understanding of where the trends are leading.

Sandra Stencel
Managing Editor

October 1983
Washington, D.C.

STAYING HEALTHY

by

Marc Leepson

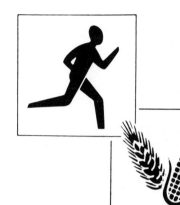

Aug. 26
1 9 8 3

STAYING HEALTHY

"YOU KNOW, DOCTOR," a 33-year-old woman said to her cardiologist, "I always try to follow my grandmother's advice and stay away from doctors as much as possible." The physician, who heads the cardiology department at a large hospital in Washington, D.C., replied: "That's very good advice."

It appears as if more Americans than ever before are trying to stay away from doctors by taking responsibility for their own health and practicing preventive medicine on a daily basis. Countless numbers of Americans are eating nutritiously, exercising, losing excessive weight, and trying to control stress, cigarette smoking, and alcohol and drug consumption. The main reason: an increasing awareness that these lifestyle changes can greatly reduce the risk of getting a host of serious diseases, especially the most common causes of death: heart disease and cancer.

"Physical health has taken on great importance in our lives and ... many of us are thinking about it almost to the point of obsession these days," said social psychologist Carin Rubenstein.[1] Said Jack Foard, chief operating officer of the Sun Valley Health Institute: "The decade of the eighties will be remembered as the decade of health and fitness where there was a real turnaround in the medical mentality of the country."[2]

This new awareness of the benefits of preventive medicine and the role patients can play in fighting disease is also shared by many physicians. It has brought about "something akin to a revolution in the theory and practice of medicine," wrote Norman Cousins in his 1979 best-seller *Anatomy of an Illness*. In the book, Cousins describes how he overcame a serious glandular illness through a mixture of non-traditional medical practices including megadoses of Vitamin C, continual positive thinking and a steady diet of laughter. Cousins, the author of 11 books and longtime editor of *Saturday Review*, now lectures on

[1] Writing in *Psychology Today*, October 1982, p. 28. Rubenstein, associate editor of the magazine, reported on a reader's survey on staying healthy to which some 25,000 persons responded. The survey results, Rubenstein commented, "suggest that many Americans who feel powerless to effect changes in their private lives find that physical health is their last bastion of personal control — something that they themselves can influence."

[2] Sun Valley Health Institute, based in Green Bay, Wis., sells preventive health programs to hospitals. Remarks by Foard and others in this report were, unless otherwise identified, made in interviews with the author conducted between July 29 and Aug. 3, 1983.

the doctor-patient relationship at the University of California at Los Angeles Medical School. He wrote that the growing popularity of preventive medicine represents an "important new mood in American medicine." Increasing numbers of doctors, Cousins wrote, are "attempting to diagnose and treat the patient in the context of all factors — work, nutrition, family, personality, emotions, environment — that figure in illness or breakdown." [3]

One reason doctors are now more willing to work with patients on nutrition, exercise and other "non-medical" matters is that since the mid-sixties epidemiological evidence has shown that the way a person lives has a direct bearing on health. According to the National Center for Health Statistics, about 70 percent of the deaths in this country in 1979 — the last year for which complete statistics are available — were due to diseases such as heart attacks, stroke and cancer that are closely linked to such things as cigarette smoking, improper diet and lack of exercise *(see table, p. 7)*. "These killers are not caused by a single bacteria or virus, but have several 'risk factors' associated with their development," said Dr. Charles A. Berry, founder and president of the National Foundation for the Prevention of Disease. "Most are lifestyle items such as smoking, fat intake, and numerous other factors." [4]

Preventive Medicine's Wide Acceptance

Evidence of the widespread acceptance of preventive medicine theories is not difficult to find. More than 2,250 hospitals now offer some type of health-promotion program, according to the American Hospital Association. Some 400 hospitals have constructed fitness facilities within the hospital grounds. The American Medical Association, which since its founding in 1846 has worked primarily to further covential, scientific medicine, now heartily endorses the preventive concept. "Major gains can still be made in reducing illness and disability through preventive measures," Dr. Joseph Boyle, chairman of the AMA's board of trustees, told Congress last spring. [5]

The AMA last year formally endorsed the practice of "medical evaluation of healthy persons." Checkups not only can help doctors detect serious diseases while they are still treatable, the AMA said, but also can give patient and physician "the opportunity to build the mutual trust and knowledge that will stand them in good stead, not only when acute illness may require the physician's care, but also when the physician at-

[3] Norman Cousins, *Anatomy of an Illness* (1979), pp. 50, 110.
[4] Writing in the Health Insurance Association of America publication, "An Approach to Good Health for Employees and Reduced Health Care Cost for Industry," p. 5.
[5] Testifying April 26, 1983, before the U.S. Senate Labor and Human Resources Committee.

HEALTH RISK FACTORS*

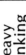

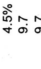
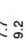
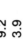
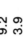

State	Obesity	Sedentary Lifestyle	High Blood Pressure	Cigarette Smoking	Heavy Drinking
Alabama	24.2%	12.3%	6.1%	30.8%	4.5%
Delaware	20.3	14.2	4.5	29.7	9.7
District of Columbia	23.7	17.4	6.0	33.0	9.7
Florida	26.3	13.1	4.0	32.2	14.5
Indiana	24.6	12.7	3.5	33.2	7.7
Kansas	21.2	9.5	3.5	23.4	9.2
Kentucky	24.9	13.5	5.1	37.1	3.9
Montana	17.9	9.7	3.3	25.9	7.5
Nebraska	23.1	11.6	3.3	24.4	5.8
New Jersey	23.6	17.4	3.7	32.0	8.9
North Carolina	26.3	13.2	5.7	37.1	4.5
Ohio	24.8	NA	3.3	32.2	3.8
Virginia	21.8	13.6	2.8	32.1	7.5
West Virginia	25.6	11.4	4.4	31.7	3.5
CALIFORNIA	24.3	9.5			

* Percentage of adults with risk factors associated with seven of the 10 leading causes of death. Source: Centers for Disease Control.

tempts to foster those behaviors and activities that contribute to the prolonging of the patient's health and productive life." [6]

One important reason for the unprecedented interest today in keeping healthy is the rapidly escalating cost of health care. Americans spent a record $321.4 billion on health care in 1982. In a year in which overall inflation increased by only 3.9 percent, health costs rose by 11 percent. Hospital costs alone went up 12.6 percent.[7] The portion of the nation's gross national product (GNP) spent on health care has risen from 6 percent in 1965 to more than 10 percent today. Some experts argue that the steep increases in medical care costs have not been accompanied by an increased quality of medical care. "We are getting less for the money than in times past," said George Crile Jr., former head of general surgery at the Cleveland Clinic. Crile noted that life expectancy rose by only about 3.3 years from 1960 to 1980, compared to 7-to-8-year increases in each of the 20-year periods from 1900 to 1960. "These figures suggest that the law of diminishing returns is beginning to operate," Crile said.[8]

Antecedents of the Wellness Concept

Preventive medicine techniques date from ancient Chinese medical texts of the 27th and 26th centuries B.C. that discussed ways of life necessary to maintain good health. Classical Greek medical scholarship also had the seeds of preventive concepts. Hippocrates, the 4th century B.C. Greek physician widely acknowledged as the father of medicine, taught that medical treatment should above all be based on building a patient's strength through proper diet and hygienic measures. According to medical writer Robert M. Cunningham Jr., the legendary Greek physician Asclepius, the son of Apollo and Coronis, "built his temples of healing for the ancient Greeks" in which "baths, diet, and exercise were as much a part of the treatment as medicines were." [9]

The biggest advances in preventive medicine came in the last half of the 19th century when doctors interested in public health managed to put widespread sanitary reforms into effect. "That's when we began getting rid of infectious diseases," said Ken Dane, director of research for the American College of Preventive Medicine. "We learned to intervene between the vector for the disease and the hosts. In the case of cholera, for example, [we intervened] between the water pump that was

---

[6] "Medical Evaluations of Healthy Persons," report of the Council on Scientific Affairs, approved by the House of Delegates of the American Medical Association, June 15, 1982. The AMA last year also established a division of personal and public health policy and has placed more emphasis on its food and nutrition program.
[7] See "Rising Cost of Health Care," *E.R.R.*, 1983 Vol. I, pp. 253-272.
[8] Writing in *The Washington Post*, July 31, 1983.
[9] Robert M. Cunningham Jr., *Wellness at Work* (1982), p. 10.

Leading Causes of Death*

Rank	Cause of Death	Percent of Total Deaths
1	Diseases of the heart	38.3
2	Cancer	21.1
3	Stroke	8.9
4	Accidents	5.5
5	Lung disease	2.6
6	Pneumonia and influenza	2.4
7	Diabetes	1.7
8	Liver disease	1.6
9	Atherosclerosis	1.5
10	Suicide	1.4

* 1979 figures

Source: National Center for Health Statistics

producing the disease and the individual by removing the pump. This was when quarantine — keeping people away from each other to prevent transmitting germs — came into being."

Another breakthrough in disease prevention came in the 1940s and 1950s when effective vaccines were developed for diseases such as poliomyelitis. Other preventive concepts, however, were not popular during that time. "During the 1950s and 1960s," a government report noted, "concern with the treatment of chronic diseases and lack of knowledge about their causes resulted in a decline in emphasis on prevention." [10] Preventive medicine concepts did not begin gaining widespread acceptance until the early 1970s.

A combination of factors is responsible for today's wide interest in preventive practices. First, beginning in the 1960s came an increased public awareness of the dangerous side effects of powerful medical drugs such as thalidomide and antibiotics. "The public's awareness of these dangers rose very sharply in the 1960s and 1970s, as consumer consciousness expanded into the health field," Norman Cousins wrote. "The result was a growing distrust not just of the highly sophisticated new drugs but of almost all medications in general." [11]

In addition, many Americans became disillusioned with the overspecialization in medicine and what was viewed as an overemphasis on impersonal technology. The distrust of powerful medications and impersonalized, overly technological medical procedures prompted new interest in the "soft" side of medicine. "Folk, non-Western and entirely novel therapies gained not only a clientele [in the 1970s], but also surprising

---

[10] "Healthy People: The Surgeon General's Report on Health Promotion and Disease Prevention," July 1979, p. 1-6.
[11] Cousins, op. cit., pp. 113-114.

respectability," wrote Harvard University sociologist Paul Starr. These new therapies presented themselves "as a humane alternative to an overly technical, disease-oriented, impersonal medical system." [12]

Another outgrowth of the public distrust of overly technical, impersonal modern medicine was a new interest in treating or preventing disease through the use of natural substances. Attention focused on nutrition and the nutritional shortcomings of the standard American diet. "Ten years ago, nutrition was kind of passed off as not being very important in health care at all," said Dave Callahan, marketing and public relations director of the American International Hospital in Zion, Ill. "Today it's becoming more and more recognized that nutrition, if not *the* central component of wellness and well-being, is certainly a very important component."

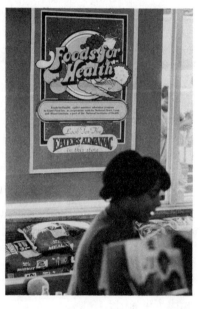

Among the factors influencing public opinion about the role of diet and health was the widespread publicity given to the conclusions of a report by the Special U.S. Senate Committee on Nutrition and Human Needs in January 1977. The report said that the typical American diet contained too much refined sugar, salt and animal fat, and recommended that Americans eat more fresh fruits, vegetables, grains and natural foods.

As nutrition became more popular, the American public became aware that the subject was not being taught in most medical schools. The fact that nutrition "had no standing of its own in most medical schools ran counter to the public's conviction that nutrition was at the very top of factors affecting health," Norman Cousins commented. There is more emphasis on nutrition in medical education today, but most American medical schools do not offer specific courses on the subject. Dr. Harold Lubin, director of the AMA's food and nutrition program, said that some medical schools have resisted implementing nutrition courses, but that there is a heightened interest in

---

[12] Paul Starr, *The Social Transformation of Modern Medicine* (1982), p. 392.

nutrition today among medical students. "They want to know that information," Lubin said. "With their interest, I think that we'll see some additional headway [in adding nutrition courses]. Strides have been made, but not to the extent that we'd like yet."

In recent years, too, there has been greater public knowledge of medical advances and the health risks associated with late 20th-century lifestyles. Many Americans first became aware of the dangers of cigarette smoking, for example, when the famous Surgeon General's Report on Smoking and Health was issued in 1964 linking cigarette smoking to several fatal or disabling diseases. A subsequent 1979 Surgeon General's Report recounted more than 24,000 scientific surveys that showed that cigarette smoking causes most cases of lung cancer and is a major factor in increasing the risk of heart attacks. The Surgeon General now categorically states that cigarette smoking "is the single most preventable cause of death" in this country.

Holistic Medicine; the 'Placebo Effect'

The final component that helped bring about today's widespread popularity of preventive techniques was an increased public awareness of the mind-body connection: the idea that the human body may not only prevent but also overcome most health problems without the use of drugs. This concept is the cornerstone of what became known as the holistic health movement of the 1970s. Dr. Jerome D. Frank of Johns Hopkins University's department of psychiatry and behavioral sciences characterized holistic medicine as viewing the human body "as an open system that seeks to preserve internal harmony among biological and psychological processes, as well as harmony between the total organism and the biological and social environment." Holistic health practitioners view disease, Dr. Frank wrote, "as perturbation of the whole system and health as harmony. Treatment is, therefore, aimed at putting the total system back into smooth functioning through working at spiritual, psychological, and social, as well as bodily levels." [13]

Holistic treatment techniques, sometimes used in conjunction with standard, scientific medical treatments, have proven successful in fighting diseases ranging from obesity to cancer. But the concept has been derided by traditional physicians who are skeptical that the body can overcome diseases without scientific medical treatment. Holistic proponents say that there is scientific proof that the mind and body are linked. They say that holistic techniques such as visualization and biofeedback can help the brain release endorphins — the body's own pain-

---

[13] Writing in *Johns Hopkins Medical Journal*, December 1981, p. 223.

suppressing chemical substances that are closely related to opiates such as morphine[14]. Holistic proponents say that since negative emotions can produce diseases such as ulcers, hypertension and stomach and bowel ailments, then positive emotions can help ward off or cure physiological problems. "Each patient carries his own doctor inside him," Dr. Albert Schweitzer once said.

Another piece of evidence that the mind and body are linked is the placebo effect in which a patient exhibits physical changes after being given a harmless, unmedicated preparation. In one clinical test a group of patients given a placebo but told they were receiving a potent cold prevention tablet (ascorbic acid) had fewer colds than a group given ascorbic acid and told they were getting a placebo. The placebo effect is "one of the most interesting phenomena in medicine," said author Stephen Jay Gould of Harvard University. "States of mind inspired by confidence clearly influence the course of healing." [15]

Placebos, Gould commented, are one reason for the effectiveness of the "old-fashioned" medical approach of doctors who develop close relationships with patients and pay close attention to their problems in a personal way. Norman Cousins wrote that the placebo effect "is proof that there is no real separation between mind and body...." [16]

Wellness Program Components

THE NEW POPULARITY of preventive medicine is changing the way many physicians define good health. In the past, doctors tended to consider the absence of disease or of any serious medical problem a clean bill of health. But today more physicians are looking beyond symptoms to other factors in determining optimal health. "We think that not only must individuals manifest no signs of diseases, but they also should have an absence of risk factors such as cigarette smoking, obesity, high blood-fat levels and totally sedentary existence — the things that have been demonstrated as significant risks for future cardiovascular disease," said Dr. William Wanago, director of medicine for Executive Health Examiners, a New York-based health service organization specializing in preventive and occupational medicine.

---

[14] For background, see "Brain Research," *E.R.R.*, 1978 Vol. II, pp. 661-680 and "Chronic Pain: The Hidden Epidemic, *E.R.R*, 1983 Vol. I, pp. 393-412.
[15] Writing in *The New York Review of Books,* July 21, 1983, pp. 11-12.
[16] Cousins, *op. cit.,* p. 56.

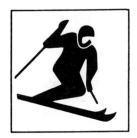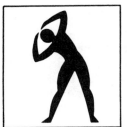

These risk factors are "asymptomatic states that people have which may lead to disease," said Ken Dane, director of research of the American College of Preventive Medicine. "Take smoking, for example. A preventive medicine practitioner, in a sense, would see you coming through the door, note the pack of Luckies in your left-hand pocket and say, 'There goes a man who is at risk for a heart attack. I don't have to wait until he's got pains in his chest to tell this man that he may have a heart attack.' Instead of focusing on the symptom — which is downstream from the precursor or risk factor — you focus on the risk factor itself. . . . They include high blood pressure, smoking, the lack of exercise, perhaps inordinate obesity and a host of other things."

Preventive practitioners' main job is to help ameliorate health risk factors. Increasing numbers of physicians in recent years have begun "prescribing" regular exercise as a way to increase overall health and reduce the risk of developing a number of serious health problems, especially cardiovascular disease.

Unprecedented numbers of Americans began undertaking regular exercise programs in this country in the 1970s.[17] The exercise boom brought physical fitness into the lives of tens of millions of men and women, from pre-teenagers to senior citizens. Skeptics viewed it as a fad popularized by young affluent adults caught up in the narcissistic pleasures of the "me-decade." But all signs now indicate that the exercise boom continues unabated today.

According to the President's Council on Physical Fitness and Sports, nearly half of all adult Americans say they exercise regularly. The American Running and Fitness Association estimates that in 1982 some 33.3 million Americans considered themselves runners or joggers. Millions of others are involved in swimming, cycling and racket sports. Among the exercise programs that have gained great numbers of new adherents in recent years are dance exercises (especially among women) and weight training regimens based on recently developed strength-building equipment such as Nautilus and Universal machines.

---

[17] See "Physical Fitness Boom," *E.R.R.*, 1978 Vol. I, pp. 261-280.

There are many reasons for the continued popularity of exercise: More adults have more leisure time than ever before. Many equate exercise with good looks, popularity and sex appeal. But the experts say that the No. 1 reason for the continued exercise boom is that most exercisers believe that their regular workout helps prevent disease and perhaps increases longevity. Numerous epidemiological and clinical studies have convinced doctors of the benefits of exercise. Exercise is now an accepted part of the rehabilitation routine for recuperating heart attack patients. Not too many years ago nearly all physicians advised recovering heart patients to take it easy, get plenty of rest and even avoid walking up stairs.

Exercise: Antidote to Sedentary Living

Doctors routinely prescribe a balanced vigorous exercise program as an antidote to the physical problems that face those who live sedentary lives. Exercise can help sedentary individuals reduce stress, lose weight and — most important — increase the efficiency of the cardiovascular system to help ward off heart disease. Dr. James Nora, director of preventive cardiology at the University of Colorado School of Medicine, described the physical dangers of the sedentary lifestyle. "The less physical work you do, the less physical work your body becomes capable of doing," Dr. Nora wrote. "And the converse is also true: The more physical work you do (up to defined limits), the more you become able to do.... Demand little and you get little. Demand a lot and you get a lot." [18]

Clinical studies have shown that aerobic exercises — the slow, steady, non-stop regimens such as jogging or running, walking, swimming and cycling — help the entire cardiovascular system work more efficiently. After several months of aerobic training, most persons experience a series of physiological changes that enable them to run, walk, cycle or swim for longer periods of time without feeling overly tired. In a sense, aerobic training builds up the heart muscles, allowing the heart to pump increased amounts of freshly oxygenated blood rapidly with each beat. The most visible evidence of an efficient cardiovascular system is resting heartbeat. With regular aerobic training, many persons experience a drop of their resting heartbeat from the average 70 to 80 beats per minute to 55 to 65. When the resting heartbeat lowers, the heart beats thousands of times fewer each day.

Exercise physicians have long suspected that continued aerobic training can help lower blood pressure. Two ongoing clinical studies have provided preliminary evidence that the theory is

---

[18] James Jackson Nora, *The Whole Heart Book* (1980), p. 156. Also see Marc Leepson, *Executive Fitness* (1983), pp. 1-14.

valid. The studies are being conducted by the Institute for Aerobics Research, founded by former Air Force physician Kenneth H. Cooper (who developed the aerobics concept in the early 1960s) and the Veterans Administration Hospital in Jackson, Miss. The studies have found that patients with mild cases of high blood pressure who take part in moderately vigorous 30-minute aerobic exercises three times a week can lower their blood pressure by 10 to 20 percent. "I think this is the first good evidence that exercise alone can lower blood pressure," said researcher John Martin of the VA hospital, who also cautioned that the results were only "preliminary." [19]

Nearly all preventive medicine programs contain an exercise "prescription." Most wellness programs, for example, work with individuals to tailor an exercise program based on physical examinations and psychological profiles. In a wellness program developed by the Sun Valley Health Institute and used in 22 hospitals across the country, each participant is examined by an exercise physiologist, a nutritionist and a psychologist. Then a personalized exercise program is drawn up. "We try to sort of custom build a lifestyle that's best for each individual," said Jack Foard, the institute's chief operating officer. "We don't try to make joggers out of everyone. We help them find the proper exercise program that fits their lifestyle and temperament."

Experts say that the ideal exercise program should have three components: some type of stretching exercise for flexibility, an aerobic exercise for the cardiovascular system, and a strength-building exercise consisting either of calisthenics or weight training. Each exercise should be undertaken at least three times a week. For aerobics, the experts recommend sessions of 20 to 30 minutes; for stretching, 10-15 minutes; and for strength building, 10-15 minutes. Some exercisers combine all three components into one 40-to-60-minute session they undertake at least three times a week.

Controlling Weight and Eating Properly

Eating correctly and maintaining proper body weight also are integral parts of preventive medicine programs. "Your diet can influence your risk of developing an imposing list of life-shortening and typically American diseases," wrote *The New York Times* personal health columnist Jane Brody. They include "heart disease, cancer, stroke, diabetes and high blood pressure, not to mention the less threatening but painful problems of tooth decay, bone fractures, and — America's leading ailment — obesity." [20] Although there is some disagreement, most experts define obesity as being at least 20 percent over

---

[19] Quoted in *USA Today*, Aug. 5, 1983.
[20] Jane Brody, *Jane Brody's Nutrition Book* (1981), p. 5.

ideal weight. About 15 percent of the adult males and some 25 percent of the adult females fit into that category; some 46 percent of all adult Americans are at least 10 percent over-weight.[21] Studies have linked obesity to high blood pressure, gall bladder disease, arthritis, diabetes and heart disease, among other problems. An obese person's excess poundage additionally puts a strain on all of the body's systems, especially the cardiovascular system. The American Heart Association and many heart specialists recognize obesity as one of the risk factors associated with heart diseases (*see box, p. 5).*

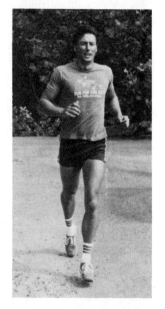

Because obesity is one health risk factor that can be controlled in most cases, preventive health practitioners offer specific programs to help patients lose weight. These programs do not promise miracle weight loss or use fad diets. Instead, preventive weight loss programs concentrate on changing eating and exercise behavior permanently to help individuals reach and maintain their ideal weight. There is a basic disagreement over how and why people lose weight. Many doctors believe that weight loss involves burning calories: If you consume more calories than you burn, you gain weight; if you burn more calories than you consume, you lose weight.

The "setpoint" theory of weight loss, on the other hand, holds that each person has an inherited biological setpoint that controls body weight because it "sets" the amount of fat in our cells. No amount of dieting can alter the setpoint. The only way to lower the setpoint is by engaging in regular exercise, especially aerobics. In this respect the setpoint theory agrees with the calorie-counting theory of weight loss which also emphasizes exercise as a way to lose weight by burning off unneeded calories.

The Providence Hospital Wellness Institute in Washington, D.C., runs a 10-week weight-reduction program based on the behavioral modification technique. Each participant in the program takes part in ten 90-minute weekly sessions. Participants consult with dieticians and nutritionists in the first session, during which body measurements are taken and each person's

---

[21] See "Weight Control: A National Obsession," *E.R.R.* 1982 Vol. II, pp. 853-868.

ideal weight is determined. During the next nine weeks participants meet and discuss eating patterns and their feelings about
food and eating. "One 'cookbook' of [weight reduction] techniques won't work for everyone," the program's promotional
brochure notes, "Therefore, the program relies heavily on individual problem-solving. Each participant learns to interpret
his or her own behavioral patterns, and devises a personal,
tailor-made behavior change program." Since June 1982 when
the weight-reduction program started, male participants have
lost an average of 19 percent of their body fat and 16 pounds.
Women have lost an average of 13.5 percent and six pounds.

Along with maintaining proper weight, preventive medicine
also stresses the importance of proper nutrition in reducing the
risk of disease. Medical research has shown that the typical
American diet — which is high in fat, sugar and calories — is
nutritionally incomplete, and can lead to a range of serious
health problems, including heart disease and cancer. Last year,
for example, a National Academy of Sciences report[22] found
"sufficient evidence" linking high fat consumption to cancer of
the breast and colon. The report recommended that Americans
eat less fat and more vegetables, fruits and whole grains.

Norman Cousins wrote that medical findings such as the link
between high fat intake and certain cancers compel doctors "to
take a complete nutritional profile of a patient as an essential
part of any examination workup." [23] Preventive medicine physicians follow that advice. But physicians generally receive little
training in nutrition in medical school. Most doctors, therefore,
follow the nutritional advice of the American Medical Association which discourages the use of vitamin and mineral supple-
ments, and stresses that eating a variety of foods daily provides
an adequate intake of vitamins and minerals for good health.

Stress Reduction; Dangers of Smoking

Nearly all doctors agree on the importance of managing stress
to maintain good health. Stress, a peculiar problem of urban
living, refers not to outside pressures that affect behavior
(which are called stressors), but to the body's response to those
pressures.[24] In moderate doses, stress serves a vital function.
Without any stimulation or challenge in life, human beings
cannot survive. It is even possible for persons to suffer from
hypostress, a condition resulting from not being stimulated
enough in daily life. What is much more common, however, is
hyperstress — the wear and tear on the body and mind resulting
from not being able to cope adequately with the stressful situa-

---

[22] National Academy of Sciences, "Diet, Nutrition, and Cancer," June 1982.
[23] Cousins, *op. cit.*, p. 121.
[24] See "Stress Management," *E.R.R.*, 1980 Vol. II, pp. 865-884.

tions in life. Those persons with hyperstress have an increased risk of suffering from a range of physiological and psychological health problems including ulcers, high blood pressure, heart disease, obesity, stomach ailments such as colitis, bowel problems such as constipation and diarrhea, migraine headaches, backaches, insomnia and depression.

Medical science has recognized the potential dangers of stress since the late 1940s. Nevertheless, many persons do not seem to know how to manage everyday stressors. Many of those unable to cope with life's pressures turn to alcohol, mood relaxant or "recreational" drugs, or cigarettes. Stress experts say that these outlets not only do not help alleviate the harmful effects of stress, but actually harm overall health. This is one reason the practitioners of preventive medicine offer stress-reduction classes which teach relaxation techniques such as meditation, yoga, self-hypnosis and biofeedback.

Because many stress problems are associated with work, "wellness" programs, which many businesses provide for their employees, include stress-reduction programs. Typically, a company-sponsored program teaches employees how stress can cause physical problems, what events in their lives add to stress and how to avoid the ill effects of stressful situations. "As is the case with alcoholism," said medical writer Robert M. Cunningham Jr., "many companies that have not yet seen fit to undertake comprehensive health promotion and physical fitness programs have nevertheless recognized the widespread incidence of stress among members of the work force and have hired or made available psychologists or counselors. . . ." [25]

Many wellness and preventive programs also offer special smoking cessation courses. Some companies with health programs even give bonuses and other financial rewards to employees who quit the habit or refrain from smoking on the job. Companies have found that smokers tend to have more absenteeism, disability and illness than non-smokers. It is now accepted in medical circles that cigarette smoking is closely linked to heart disease, cancer, and other serious medical problems. Dr. William Pollin, director of the National Institute on Drug Abuse, has said cigarette smoking "causes more illness and death than all other drugs." [26] Since 1964, when the surgeon general issued his warning, the proportion of young adult smokers has dropped steadily. Nevertheless, more than 56 million Americans continue to smoke cigarettes.[27]

---

[25] Cunningham, *op. cit.*, pp. 50-51.
[26] Writing in *World Smoking & Health*, a publication of the American Cancer Society, summer 1983, p. 2.
[27] See "More Adults Are Quitting Smoking," in the National Center for Health Statistics report, *Health: United States, 1982*, December 1982, pp. 26-27.

New Wellness Practitioners

ALTERNATIVE health care based on preventive medical concepts has taken hold across the country in the last decade. The first specialized program to use the term "wellness," Dr. John Travis' Wellness Resource Center, opened its doors in 1974 in Marin County, Calif., north of San Francisco. Since then, hundreds of thousands of Americans have taken part in many different types of preventive medicine offered by wellness centers, holistic health practitioners and health promotion programs. Preventive programs are now run by hospitals, businesses and non-licensed health educators. There is even an entire hospital devoted primarily to preventive medicine and the wellness concept.

The American International Hospital in Zion, Ill., north of Chicago, was founded in 1976 by businessman Richard Stephenson. The 95-bed hospital, formerly a community hospital,"is involved in an alternative-plus-traditional approach to modern health care," said Dave Callahan, the hospital's marketing and public relations director. "We combine programs and therapies which you find in a traditional hospital with alternative therapies. We are involved in the nutritional aspects of health care, as well as preventive medicine and some alternative therapies for illnesses such as cancer and cardiovascular disease."

The hospital's menu features fresh fruit and vegetables and whole grain breads. The kitchen uses honey or fructose rather than sugar, does not serve foods containing artificial colors or preservatives and offers organic foods, and vegetarian and other special diets. Family members are permitted to visit patients as frequently as possible. Callahan said that patients come to the hospital from "all over the country and all over the world." The reason, he said, is that there "is a crying need out there for this sort of health care.... More people are concerned with their health, with preventive medicine, with what one does once one becomes sick and who you go to when you are ill. It used to be that you had a family doctor and you entrusted your entire being to that person.... But nowadays people are more questioning and they're more particular about these sorts of things, especially when it comes to a dread disease such as cancer."

Hospitals' Health Promotion Programs

More and more traditional hospitals are adding health promotion and wellness programs to their normal activities. Houston's Methodist Hospital, for example, has a health-food restaurant in addition to its traditional hospital-style cafeteria. Providence Hospital in Washington, D.C., started a wellness institute in June 1982. The program originally provided hospital employees with preventive medical services. Then it began offering the same services to individuals and businesses.

The Providence Wellness Institute's basic program focuses on exercise, stress management, nutrition and preventive techniques for coronary health. Each participant first undergoes a two-day health assessment in which such things as blood pressure, resting heart rate, cholesterol and blood-fat levels are measured. The participant also provides a detailed medical history, and undergoes strength, flexibility and stress tests.

Then the institute's staff comes up with a profile showing each participant's strengths and weaknesses. After this health assessment comes a 16-hour program during which the staff works with each participant. "We help individuals focus on ways to make changes in their scores, or to maintain them if they're good and to develop their own personal plans for achieving a higher level of health," said Linda Harmon, the institute's general manager. The institute offers specific programs on weight management, smoking cessation, stress management and nutrition. It has five exercise programs: aerobic dance, gentle movement, rebounding, running/jogging/walking and pre- and post-natal exercise.

Business Interest in Healthy Workers

In the last 10 to 15 years, hundreds of companies across the country have set up their own health promotion, preventive medicine or wellness programs for employees. They want their employees to stay healthy, and thus productive. But there is still another reason. Businesses have found that preventive programs can help cut operating costs; employers pay about half of the nation's health care bill in the form of health insurance. "Healthy employees and those programs that promote their health can help reduce the trend toward ever increasing health benefit costs, absenteeism and decreased productivity," said Dr. Charles A. Berry of the National Foundation for the Prevention of Disease. "The numerous advantages of health promotion programs at the work site lead to high voluntary participation levels . . . and to benefits to the company evidenced in improved employee health and reduced overall costs." [28]

Many large corporations have multifaceted wellness programs. Kimberly-Clark Corp.'s Health Management Program, for example, provides an extensive medical screening for employees. It includes filling out a 40-page medical history

[28] Charles A. Berry, *op. cit.*, p. 5

chart, undergoing a series of laboratory tests and a treadmill exercise test. The program offers nutrition counseling, smoking cessation, blood pressure control and weight reduction programs. The company stresses physical fitness; it has spent more than $2.5 million on fitness facilities since the health management program began in October 1977. The company offers employees a 100-meter indoor running track, an Olympic-size swimming pool, an exercise room, a sauna, a whirlpool and locker room facilities.

The Times Publishing Co. in St. Petersburg, Fla., which publishes the *St. Petersburg Times* and the *Evening Independent*, started a wellness program in January 1982. The program provides staffers, retirees and family members with extensive health screenings and a series of preventive health programs. These include the standard smoking cessation, weight reduction, stress management and exercise programs, as well as such special seminars as a four-week class using biofeedback to help manage stress.

Wellness program coordinator Diane Constantino said the company decided to start a preventive program primarily because of rising health insurance costs. "Claims had gone up 90 percent over the last five years," she said. "When we looked closely we found that the root of the problem is lifestyle oriented — whether it's ulcers or high blood pressure or whatever. We decided that it was time to do something positive, something preventive." The company estimates that it has saved $200,000 in health insurance costs in the 18 months the program has been in operation.

Larger corporations have reported even bigger savings. New York Telephone, for example, which employs 80,000 persons, estimated that nine of its wellness programs saved some $2.7 million in absences and treatment costs in 1980. The company also reported other, non-monetary measures of success with the programs. Some 57 percent of those who went through the smoking cessation program, for example, were able to quit their habit; 79 percent of the 5,200 employees who had high blood pressure were able to bring it under control; and 25 lives were saved through early detection of lung disease and cancer.

If lives continue to be saved, health improved and health costs cut, there is little doubt that preventive medicine and wellness programs will continue to remain popular. Another factor is the public's interest. "Many more people are probably interested in aspects of health care than I suspect at any time in our history," said Dr. Harold Lubin of the AMA's food and nutrition program. If that interest continues, the preventive medicine and wellness movements also will continue to thrive.

Selected Bibliography

Books

Brody, Jane, *Jane Brody's Nutrition Book: A Lifetime Guide to Good Eating for Better Health and Weight Control*, Norton, 1981.

Cousins, Norman, *Anatomy of an Illness as Perceived by the Patient*, Norton, 1979.

Cunningham, Robert M. Jr., *Wellness at Work*, Inquiry, 1982.

Eckholm, Erik P., *The Picture of Health: Environmental Sources of Disease*, Norton, 1977.

Leepson, Marc, *Executive Fitness*, McGraw-Hill, 1983.

Selye, Hans, *The Stress of Life*, McGraw-Hill, 1956.

Starr, Paul, *The Social Transformation of American Medicine*, Basic Books, 1982.

Thomas, Lewis, *The Youngest Science: Notes of a Medicine Watcher*, Viking, 1983.

Articles

"Advance Report of Final Mortality Statistics," *NCHS* [National Center for Health Statistics] *Monthly Vital Statistics Report*, Sept. 30, 1982.

American Cancer Society Journal, selected issues.

American Health, selected issues.

Celarier, Michelle, "Big Bucks in the Wellness Biz," *Ms.*, May 1983.

Frank, Jerome D. "Holistic Medicine — A View From the Fence," *The Johns Hopkins Medical Journal*, December 1981.

Rubenstein, Carin, "Wellness is All," *Psychology Today*, October 1982.

"The Concept of Health as Wellness," *The Center Magazine*, January-February 1983.

White, Philip L. and Nancy Selvey, "Nutrition and the New Health Awareness," *Journal of the American Medical Association*, June 4, 1982.

Reports and Studies

American Medical Association, Division of Scientific Analysis and Technology, "Medical Evaluations of Healthy Persons," 1983.

Berry, Charles A., "An Approach to Good Health for Employees & Reduced Health Care Costs for Industry," Health Insurance Association of America, 1981.

Editorial Research Reports: "Rising Cost of Health Care," 1983 Vol. I, p. 253; "Stress Management," 1980 Vol. II, p. 865; "Physical Fitness Boom," 1978 Vol. I, p. 261.

President's Council on Physical Fitness and Sports, "An Introduction to Physical Fitness," 1982; "How Different Sports Rate in Promoting Physical Fitness," 1978.

U.S. Department of Health and Human Services, "Health, United States, 1982," December 1982.

U.S. Public Health Service, Office of the Assistant Secretary for Health and Surgeon General, "Healthy People: The Surgeon General's Report on Health Promotion and Disease Prevention," July 1979.

Photos: p. 8 by U.S. Department of Agriculture; p. 14 by Marc Leepson.

Rising cost of health care

by

Mary H. Cooper and Sandra Stencel

Apr. 8
1 9 8 3

21

Editor's Note: Detailed rules outlining a new system for reimbursing hospitals for treating Medicare patients were made public by the Reagan administration on Aug. 31, 1983. The prospective reimbursement plan, which uses predetermined rates for all patients with the same illness or injury, was approved by Congress in March 1983 *(see p. 26)*. The administration supported the measure as a means of bringing health care costs under control.

Another of Reagan's cost-containment proposals was rejected Aug. 24 by the Advisory Council on Social Security, a year-old committee set up by the Department of Health and Human Services to study proposals aimed at keeping Medicare's hospital insurance trust fund afloat in coming years. The panel, chaired by former Indiana Gov. Otis R. Bowen, a Republican, rejected the president's proposal to make employers' contributions to group health insurance plans, now a tax-free fringe benefit, taxable to participating employees *(see p. 28)*.

Another administration proposal, which would increase the amount the program's elderly beneficiaries must pay for short-term hospital stays, is widely viewed as too hot a political issue for Congress to tackle — or the White House to push — before the 1984 presidential election *(see p. 29)*.

RISING COST OF HEALTH CARE

FOR Americans hard pressed by double-digit unemployment and high interest rates, one of the few encouraging developments during the current recession has been a fall in the rate of inflation. In 1982, the Consumer Price Index (CPI) rose by a relatively low 3.9 percent, five points below the 1981 figure.[1] But one component of the index continued to climb at a faster rate than other consumer prices. The amount Americans spent on health care in 1982 rose 11 percent over the previous year to a record $321.4 billion; hospital costs alone rose 12.6 percent last year. And while consumer prices actually fell by 0.2 percent in February 1983, medical costs went up 0.8 percent. The portion of the nation's gross national product (GNP) spent on health care has risen from 6 percent in 1965 to 10 percent today.

The federal government's contribution to the nation's health care bill also continues to climb, as rising hospital and physicians' charges are reflected in the cost of Medicare, Medicaid and other public health programs. Combined outlays for Medicare, the federal health care program for the elderly, and Medicaid, the state-federal program for the poor and disabled, are projected to reach $75 billion in fiscal 1983, accounting for 9.5 percent of the federal budget.

President Reagan has described the rate of increase in health care costs as "excessive," undermining "people's ability to purchase needed health care."[2] To help bring health costs under control, the administration has proposed a series of reform measures reflecting the president's often stated goal of reducing government influence and restoring public services to the private sector. One of these measures — a plan to set up a new system for reimbursing hospitals for treating Medicare patients — was approved by Congress March 25 as part of the Social Security rescue bill *(see p. 26)*.[3]

Among the other cost-containment proposals Reagan sent Congress was one to set up a voucher system expanding "oppor-

---

[1] Published monthly by the Department of Labor's Bureau of Labor Statistics, the CPI follows a "market basket" of goods and services and determines the rate of price variation for each over the previous month.
[2] Message on his proposed budget for fiscal 1984, delivered to Congress Jan. 31, 1983.
[3] For background on the Social Security system's financial problems, see "Social Security Options," *E.R.R.*, 1982 Vol. II, pp. 929-948.

tunities for Medicare beneficiaries to use their benefits to enroll
in private health plans as an alternative to traditional Medicare
coverage." Reagan also asked Congress to begin taxing em-
ployer-sponsored health insurance benefits *(see p. 28)* and to
require Medicare beneficiaries to pay more out of their own
pockets for short-term hospital stays. This plan would be cou-
pled with "catastrophic" coverage for long illnesses *(see p. 29)*.
Reagan also proposed that Medicaid beneficiaries be required to
pay nominal fees of $1 to $2 for each visit to a doctor or hospital.
Under current law, states may impose such "cost-sharing" re-
quirements, but are not required to do so.[4]

While the administration's health care reform package was
presented as a cost-control initiative, the projected savings
would be relatively small, at least in the short term. The
Department of Health and Human Services estimated that the
package would save $4.2 billion in fiscal 1984. But even if all the
proposals are enacted, federal outlays for health would increase
nearly 10 percent in fiscal 1984, to $90.6 billion, from the 1983
level of $82.4 billion, according to the budget.

The Factors Behind Health Care Inflation

The reasons for mounting health care costs are varied and
complex. They include such things as the growing size and age
of the elderly population, higher salaries for nurses and other
hospital workers, and the increase in the number of malpractice
suits, which many believe has caused doctors to overtreat their
patients in an effort to protect themselves from possible legal
action.

Consumer expectations were regarded as a primary cause of
the problem in a recent survey of health experts conducted by
Yankelovich, Skelly and White, Inc., for *Prevention* magazine.[5]
One reason for consumers' "nearly limitless expectations of the
system," the report said, was the fact that the cost of medical
treatment has to a great extent been shifted to third parties.
Patients pay only 29 percent of the nation's health care bill out
of their own pockets, not enough, critics say, to make them cost-
conscious. Public funds, including Medicare and Medicaid, pay
42 percent of the nation's medical costs, while private insurance
companies cover 27 percent *(see box, p. 27)*. Both private and
public insurance plans reimburse health care providers on a fee-
for-service basis for "reasonable" costs incurred in the treatment of beneficiaries, a system that many believe offers neither

---

[4] For additional information on Reagan's proposals, see *Congressional Quarterly Weekly
Report*, Feb. 5, 1983, pp. 275-278.
[5] "The American Health System: A Survey of Leaders and Experts," March 1983. Copies
of the report may be obtained from the Market Services Dept., *Prevention Magazine*,
Rodale Press, Inc., 33 East Minor Street, Emmaus, Pa. 18049.

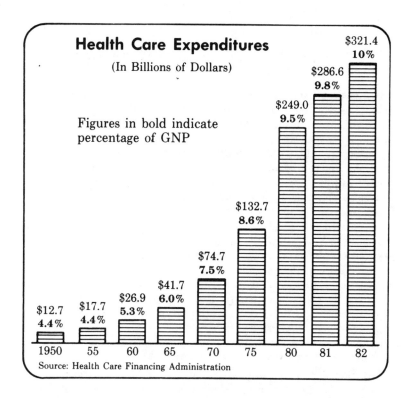

Health Care Expenditures

(In Billions of Dollars)

Figures in bold indicate
percentage of GNP

$321.4
10%

$286.6
9.8%

$249.0
9.5%

$132.7
8.6%

$74.7
7.5%

$41.7
6.0%

$26.9
5.3%

$12.7
4.4%

$17.7
4.4%

1950   55   60   65   70   75   80   81   82

Source: Health Care Financing Administration

physicians nor hospital administrators any incentive to control costs; essentially, the more they charge, the more they make.

Another factor behind rising health care costs has to do with advances in medical technology that entail expensive equipment, such as the sophisticated X-ray device called a computerized axial tomography (CAT) scanner, or complicated surgical procedures such as coronary bypass operations and organ transplants. Other innovative hospital services, such as intensive care units and kidney dialysis machines, also entail high per-patient charges. The suggestion that such services be used with greater discretion in the interest of controlling costs has stirred intense debate over the moral implications of applying "cost-benefit" analysis to decisions regarding human life.

Administration's 'Free-Market' Strategy

Throughout the 1970s, much of the debate over reform of the health care delivery system centered on various proposals for national health insurance (see p. 34). After the election of Ronald Reagan, however, the focus of debate shifted to the president's calls for a "pro-competitive" or "free-market" health policy.[6] The president's goal was to make health care

[6] For background, see "Reagan Seeks 'Competition' in U.S. Health Care System," *Congressional Quarterly Weekly Report,* Feb. 20, 1982, pp. 331-333.

providers and their patients more cost-conscious by making them more aware of the full costs of medical care.

In his first two years in office, Reagan succeeded in reducing federal spending for health programs and in turning over responsibility for many of them to the states. Cost-reduction measures in the budget reconciliation laws of 1981 and 1982 included (1) a 25 percent increase in the amount elderly Medicare recipients had to pay for medical care; and (2) consolidation of funding for such programs as community health centers, drug and alcohol abuse centers, and maternal and child health programs into four block grants. The states then assumed responsibility for allocating the funds according to federal guidelines. The administration's changes allowed the states greater flexibility in the administration of Medicaid, and according to a recent article in *The New England Journal of Medicine,* more than 30 states have cut back spending on this health care assistance program for the poor by reducing benefits, tightening eligibility standards or simply cutting reimbursements to health care programs.[7]

Prospective Reimbursement for Medicare

On Dec. 28, 1982, the Department of Health and Human Services (HHS) sent Congress a report outlining the administration's plan for replacing the existing Medicare reimbursement system, under which charges are calculated after services have been rendered, with a "prospective" system that would set prices in advance. The administration was required to come up with the plan under the terms of the 1982 tax bill, approved by Congress on Aug. 19 of that year, which also placed caps on the overall amount of Medicare reimbursement.[8]

The HHS report outlined a method of using medical and financial data to assign an average price for treating 467 specific medical conditions or combinations of conditions, known as "diagnosis related groups" or DRGs. By providing for fixed payment rates in advance, the new system would end the existing policy of paying hospitals whatever it costs them to treat beneficiaries. The idea is to encourage hospitals to minimize use of expensive procedures, equipment and personnel so that their operating costs do not exceed the set prices. Hospitals that provide treatment for less than the set amount can keep the difference.

According to President Reagan, this plan will "establish

---

[7] John K. Iglehart, "The Reagan Record on Health Care," *The New England Journal of Medicine,* Jan. 27, 1983.
[8] For details on the Medicare provisions of the 1982 tax bill, see *Congressional Quarterly Weekly Report,* Aug. 21, 1982, p. 2042.

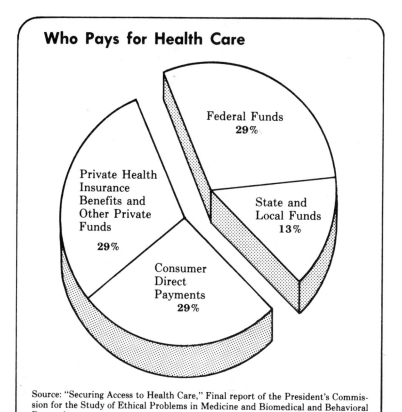

Who Pays for Health Care

Federal Funds
29%

Private Health
Insurance
Benefits and
Other Private
Funds

29%

State and
Local Funds
13%

Consumer
Direct
Payments
29%

Source: "Securing Access to Health Care," Final report of the President's Commission for the Study of Ethical Problems in Medicine and Biomedical and Behavioral Research.

Medicare as a prudent buyer of services and will ensure for both hospitals and the federal government a predictable payment for services. . . . Medicare traditionally paid hospitals . . . whatever they spent. There were, therefore, weak incentives for hospitals to conserve costs and operate efficiently." Under the new plan, he said, " hospitals with higher costs will not be able to pass on extra costs to Medicare beneficiaries and thus will face strong incentives to make cost-effective changes in practices." [9]

The administration's plan, with some modifications, was approved by the House Ways and Means Committee on March 2. To help speed its approval, the committee attached the plan to a bill for overhauling the Social Security system. That bill was approved by Congress March 25 and sent to the president for signing.

Unlike the administration's original proposal, which called for setting one national price for each ailment, the bill approved by Congress allows for regional cost differences and differences between rural and urban hospitals. The bill also would provide

[9] Message sending his health incentives reform program to Congress, Feb. 28, 1983.

exceptions for special high-cost hospitals, such as research and teaching hospitals, and would allow Medicare to make extra payments in special cases where people required extra care.

One reason the bill passed so quickly was that it had the support of influential hospital lobbyists and two major hospital groups, the American Hospital Association (AHA) and the Federation of American Hospitals. Both preferred it to the stringent Medicare payment caps enacted as part of the 1982 tax bill. "Prospective payment will change the incentives in the health system and allow hospital administrators to better manage their payments," a spokeswoman for AHA said in a recent interview.

The main objection to the proposal was that it would apply only to Medicare payments. Critics, including the American Association of Retired Persons and the Health Insurance Association of America,[10] claimed that in order to be effective, the DRG-based prepayment system should apply to Medicaid, private health insurance plans and individuals, as well as Medicare. Otherwise, they said, hospitals might shift the cost of providing services for Medicare recipients to private insurance companies, which would then pass on the higher charges to their subscribers through higher premiums. "Until we can solve the cost-shifting problem," said John K. Kittredge, executive vice president of The Prudential Insurance Co., "we will not have cost containment."

Officials are not sure exactly how much money will be saved by the prospective reimbursement program, which will be phased in over a three-year period, but they do not expect it to solve Medicare's mounting financial problems. A recent study by the Congressional Budget Office predicted that Medicare's Hospital Insurance Trust Fund, which is part of the Social Security system, could go broke as early as 1987.[11] The main reason for the projected deficits, according to the study, is the fact that "hospital costs are growing much more rapidly than the earnings to which the Hospital Insurance tax is applied." From 1982 to 1995, costs incurred by Medicare recipients are projected to increase by an average of 13.2 percent, while covered earnings are expected to rise by an average of only 6.8 percent over the same period.

Opposition to Health Insurance Tax Plan

President Reagan's other proposals for curbing health care costs are more controversial than the Medicare reimbursement plan. Particularly controversial is his plan to tax part of em-

---

[10] Both the American Association of Retired Persons and the Health Insurance Association of America are located in Washington, D.C.
[11] Congressional Budget Office, "Prospects for Medicare's Hospital Insurance Trust Fund," February 1983.

ployer-provided health insurance benefits. The administration contends that under current law neither employees nor employers have much incentive to hold down costs. Company-sponsored benefits represent tax-free income to employees and tax-deductible business expenses to employers.

The administration wants to change this arrangement by putting a ceiling on the amount of insurance premium payments that would continue to receive preferential tax treatment. It would require employees to pay taxes on employer contributions to their health insurance in excess of $175 a month for family coverage or $70 a month for individual coverage. The administration believes this would encourage employees to pressure employers for less comprehensive insurance coverage. The average yearly income tax increase for each of the 16.5 million Americans currently receiving employer-provided health insurance benefits above the proposed ceiling would be about $140, according to administration estimates.

Reagan's proposal elicits stiff resistance from organized labor. The AFL-CIO Executive Council said the proposed tax would constitute "an unprecedented intrusion in collective bargaining" that would "turn back the clock on decades of progress by workers in winning comprehensive health care protection." [12] Organized labor is not alone in its opposition. Representatives of about 50 groups, ranging from the Chamber of Commerce of the United States and the National Association of Manufacturers to the National Council of Senior Citizens, met with Sen. Bob Packwood, R-Ore., in early January to voice their opposition to the plan. Packwood told them there was "no constituency" for the tax scheme and predicted its defeat. He said such a plan would erode the health of working Americans and set a precedent for taxes on other fringe benefits.

Controversy Over Other Reagan Proposals

Also controversial is Reagan's suggestion that Medicare beneficiaries pay more for short-term hospital stays. Under current law, Medicare recipients pay a deductible ($350 in fiscal 1984) for the first day of every hospital stay, but are fully covered by Medicare for the next 59 days. Coverage is only partial for the next 30 days, during which time the patient must pay 25 percent of the deductible ($87.50 per day). If the patient is hospitalized longer than three months, he has only 60 remaining "lifetime reserve days," for which he must pay one-half the deductible ($175 per day). Thereafter, the patient is personally liable for all hospital costs.

Under Reagan's plan the emphasis of Medicare coverage

---

[12] *AFL-CIO News*, March 5, 1983.

Recession's Impact on Access to Health Care

When workers are laid off or fired, they frequently lose more than just their jobs. They may also lose company-provided health insurance benefits. The Congressional Budget Office estimated that 10.7 million unemployed Americans and their families had no health insurance coverage last year.

As Congress debates the Reagan administration proposals for containing health care costs, support is building for some kind of health benefits program aimed at the unemployed. While business interests are opposed to extending health insurance benefits to the unemployed beyond the usual 30-day limit after layoff, the AFL-CIO has called for their extension for at least 65 weeks. Senate Finance Committee Chairman Robert Dole, R-Kan., has suggested that medical benefits for the unemployed could be financed with revenues collected through the administration's proposed tax on employer-provided group health insurance *(see p. 28)*.

would shift to long-term hospital stays. In addition to the full first-day deductible, Medicare recipients would pay 8 percent ($28 per day) through day 15, then 5 percent ($17.50 per day) through day 60, but receive full and unlimited coverage after that time. While the administration proposal would seem to satisfy previous calls for "catastrophic" insurance to cover long-term hospitalization, it would in fact save the government an estimated $2 billion a year, since most Medicare recipients would end up paying more for hospital care. Only about 200,000 of the 7 million Medicare recipients hospitalized each year stay longer than 60 days. The average stay is 11 days. If Reagan's plan is enacted, an 11-day hospital stay would cost Medicare beneficiaries almost twice as much as it does now.

Critics say Reagan's proposal violates the federal government's commitment to the elderly embodied in Medicare legislation. According to Janet Myder of the National Council of Senior Citizens,[13] it would impose "a very, very heavy burden" on the elderly "which is not going to be alleviated by [Reagan's proposal for] catastrophic protection. This is not catastrophic insurance. What is catastrophic for the elderly is the cost of a nursing home, the cost of any long-term care, the cumulative cost of all the things that Medicare doesn't pay for, like prescription drugs." Myder and other critics also fear that the proposed changes would lead private insurance companies to substantially increase premiums for "Medigap" policies, which pay the difference between public coverage and hospital

[13] The National Council of Senior Citizens, located at 925 15th St., N.W., Washington, D.C. 20005, represents over 4.5 million elderly people in all the states.

charges. While 60 percent of those eligible for Medicare now subscribe to private "Medigap" policies, many could no longer afford such coverage if premium prices sharply increased.

Spokesmen for groups representing the elderly also are unhappy about the administration's new interpretation of Medicaid laws, which gave states the go-ahead to require adult children of nursing home patients to pay part of the cost of their parents' care. A few states already have adopted such "family responsibility" laws, but they have delayed enforcing them awaiting federal guidelines. Rep. Henry A. Waxman, D-Calif., chairman of the House Energy and Commerce Subcommittee on Health, which has jurisdiction over Medicaid, says the administration's directive is contrary to the intent of Congress and he plans to hold hearings on the matter.

Past Approaches to Problem

THE PUBLIC and private health insurance arrangements that are partly to blame for today's health care inflation are a product of the progressive monopolization of the health care delivery system. This trend began in the latter years of the 19th century with the licensing of physicians. With fewer doctors authorized to practice medicine, fees began to rise until, by the 1920s, physicians' incomes began to far outstrip those of other workers.

Growing recognition of the impact of rising medical costs led to the formation in 1926 of the privately funded Committee on the Costs of Medical Care, which provided the first analyses of the problem in the United States and which recommended in its final reports of 1932 an increase in access to medical care for the entire population and an increase in resources to fund it. The committee's recommendations of fostering group practice and group payment for medical care were, however, condemned by the increasingly influential American Medical Association (AMA) as a dangerous challenge to the private physician's control over services provided — and fees charged — to patients. The controversy that ensued led President Franklin D. Roosevelt to exclude health care reform from the New Deal social legislation that culminated in the Social Security Act of 1935.

During the same period, both the American Hospital Association and the AMA introduced their own private insurance mechanisms, Blue Cross and Blue Shield, respectively, in response to growing demand from consumers for some form of protection from debilitating health care expenses and also to prevent single-hospital plans and prepaid group practices from weakening their monopoly of the health care delivery system. In 1934, commercial insurance companies began offering health insurance on the same fee-for-service basis, which posed few, if any, limits on the amount physicians or hospitals could charge. In this way, wrote Paul Starr, "the structure of private health plans, it seems fair to say, was basically an accommodation to provider interests." [14]

By 1958, almost two-thirds of the population was covered by hospital insurance. But while more and more Americans came under various insurance plans, only half of those aged 65 or older were covered, even though they were the most vulnerable to disease and generally the least able to pay for health care services. Awareness of the plight of the aged and poor grew throughout the 1950s and early 1960s and led to the enactment in 1965 of the Medicare and Medicaid programs.

With Medicare, all Americans, regardless of income level, are entitled upon reaching age 65 to hospital benefits as well as a voluntary supplemental policy covering 80 percent of physicians' fees. Unlike Medicare, which is funded entirely at the federal level, Medicaid was introduced as a joint state-federal program. Coverage is less uniform under this program, as the federal government may only establish standards for the types of services offered, but not the payment levels provided by the states.

Statistics indicate that Medicare and Medicaid have succeeded in greatly increasing the access of elderly and poor Americans to health care. The frequency of physician visits by people whose family incomes were below $7,000 increased by almost 50 percent between 1964 and 1980.[15] The elderly have benefited from both programs; 95 percent of them are entitled to Medicare hospital insurance, while Medicaid helps the elderly poor pay for services not covered by Medicare, such as nursing home care. In 1978, the latest year for which official statistics have been compiled, elderly Americans incurred an average annual health bill of $2,026, 63 percent of which was covered by public funds.[16]

The number of health care providers greatly increased in the 1960s, thanks largely to federal grants, scholarships and loans for medical research and education. The number of active physicians increased by 70 percent between 1965 and 1975, while the number of dentists rose by 50 percent and the number of

---

[14] Paul Starr, *The Social Transformation of American Medicine* (1982), p. 309.
[15] Department of Health and Human Services, Public Health Service, "Health, United States, 1982," p. 90.
[16] *Ibid.*, p. 152.

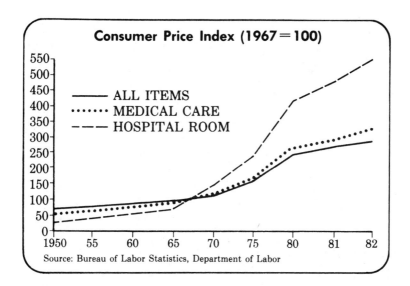

Consumer Price Index (1967 = 100)

——— ALL ITEMS
• • • • • • MEDICAL CARE
– – – HOSPITAL ROOM

Source: Bureau of Labor Statistics, Department of Labor

nurses doubled.[17] The same period saw a burst of hospital construction and expansion, with the help of federal funds provided through the Hill-Burton program, which began in 1946.

The portion of health care expenditures paid by third parties also increased during this period, rising from 45 percent in 1965 to 65 percent in 1970. In addition to Medicare and Medicaid, a major contributing factor to this trend was the inclusion of health insurance benefits in labor contracts. These group health insurance schemes benefited not only American workers, but also the health care industry itself, which no longer had to wait long periods for payment of fees.

'70s Health Care 'Crisis'; Turn to HMOs

Growing awareness of the medical inflation problem in the early 1970s led the Nixon administration to speak of a "crisis" in health care financing. Liberals and conservatives alike agreed on the need for reform of the health care system, but they disagreed on the best way to approach the problem. While liberals like Sen. Edward M. Kennedy, D-Mass., tended to favor some form of national health insurance, the Nixon administration lent its support to the increasingly popular prepaid group health plans, or health maintenance organizations (HMOs), which had first appeared as a radical alternative to the traditional control exercised over the industry by hospitals and private physicians.

The HMO evolved along two principal models. So-called "group models" operate their own facilities and employ their

---

[17] Louise B. Russell, "Medical Care," in *Setting National Priorities: Agenda for the 1980s*, ed. Joseph A. Pechman (1980), p. 175.

own physicians, nurses and other personnel. Subscribers select a primary care physician from the staff and are required to go to the group facility to receive care. With the exception of certain emergency procedures, any medical care obtained outside the facility is not covered. "Individual practice associations," on the other hand, are more decentralized. Subscribers choose a participating physician in the community, often on the basis of geographical proximity, and go to his or her office for treatment rather than to a central facility.

The HMO, by operating on a strictly prepaid basis, was seen as an effective means of encouraging physicians and hospitals to hold down costs. Since they have to work within a fixed budget, HMO physicians are unlikely to extend their patients' hospital stays beyond the time necessary for treatment. In New Jersey, for example, the average hospital stay for surgical patients enrolled in HMOs is three days, compared to four days for the general population.

Nixon's support for HMOs led to passage of a 1973 law requiring all businesses with more than 25 employees to include at least one HMO among the health benefits offered to employees. Partly as a result of this measure, the number of HMOs in the country rose from 30 in 1971 to 268 by mid-1982. The main benefit of the HMO has been a reduction in health care costs through reduced utilization of hospital services. But while effective in the communities where they exist, HMOs have yet to have a significant impact on the national health care system, as only 5 percent of the U.S. population are currently enrolled in this type of program.

National Insurance Debate; State Plans

Advocates of national health insurance were bolstered by the election of Jimmy Carter in 1976. During the presidential campaign Carter promised to introduce a "comprehensive national health insurance system with universal and mandatory coverage." But when Carter finally unveiled his plan in 1979, it turned out to be a much more limited plan to protect Americans against catastrophic medical costs. By focusing on catastrophic coverage, Carter alienated Sen. Kennedy, who was still pushing for a more comprehensive national health program similar to those available in Britain, Canada and other industrialized countries.[18]

Neither Carter's nor Kennedy's bill was approved by Congress, however, in part because of an intense lobbying campaign against them by groups representing health care providers and

---

[18] For background, see Edward M. Kennedy, *In Critical Condition: The Crisis in America's Health Care* (1972).

also because of concern in Congress over their costs. The concept of national health insurance continues to find support, particularly among organized labor and groups representing the poor and elderly. But budgetary considerations appear to have pushed this option to the back burner for the foreseeable future.

While the federal government was having trouble coming up with ways to control rising health care costs, a number of states introduced their own cost-control schemes. Some set up public agencies to review hospital budgets and/or rates, while others set up systems to regulate hospital reimbursements. Under these plans, hospitals are reimbursed prospectively in one of two ways. Either they are paid a certain rate per case of a certain type of ailment or a general budget constraint is imposed. Six states — Connecticut, Maryland, Massachusetts, New Jersey, New York and Washington — introduced prospective payment plans in 1976 or earlier. These state plans were the subject of a study that found them to be effective in containing hospital costs.[19]

It was in New Jersey that the "diagnosis-related group" (DRG) basis for calculating hospital costs was first implemented in 1980. The New Jersey plan served as the model for the new Medicare reimbursement plan recently adopted by Congress as part of the Social Security rescue bill *(see p. 26)*. Under the plan, each New Jersey hospital was required to break down all business into the 467 DRGs contained in a classification system developed at Yale University, and assign an average charge for each DRG. Patients were then billed according to their illnesses instead of the services actually received. On the basis of the hospitals' own estimates, the state of New Jersey established working annual budgets for each institution. Hospitals were encouraged to save money, as they pocketed all funds saved by working within the budget limits. But unlike the new federal program, the New Jersey plan does not just apply to Medicare, which prevents hospitals from shifting the costs incurred by some payers to other groups.

Prospects and Alternatives

C ORPORATE executives are also getting more involved in attempts to hold down health care costs. In fact, according to the report prepared by Yankelovich, Skelly and White for *Prevention* magazine, "large corporations will lead the way" in

---

[19] Brian Biles et al., "Hospital Cost Inflation Under State Rate-Setting Programs," *The New England Journal of Medicine,* Sept. 18, 1980.

solving the problem.[20] The reason for their concern is obvious. The corporate contribution to payments for health benefit plans was an estimated $60 billion in 1980. "Since World War II the employer, through negotiated benefits, has been paying more and more of the health care costs of this country for their employees and their dependents," Boyd Thompson, executive vice president of the American Association of Foundations for Medical Care, said in a recent interview. "This money was managed by insurance companies and Blue Cross-Blue Shield with no incentive on their part to hold down costs. The more the premium went up, the more money they made. Now the employers, individually and collectively, are telling the insurance companies and the Blues: 'Get out of our way, we're going to handle this ourselves by dealing with the provider directly.'"

"Since World War II the employer, through negotiated benefits, has been paying more and more of the health care costs of this country for their employees and their dependents."

Boyd Thompson, executive vice president, American Association of Foundations for Medical Care

---

In some communities corporations are banding together to form "preferred provider organizations." Under this arrangement, groups of physicians or hospitals are enlisted by employers to provide services at competitive prices. In return, the companies encourage their workers to use the services of the "preferred providers." Other companies are encouraging workers to join health maintenance organizations *(see p. 33)*. According to a newsletter published by the Group Health Association of America, Chrysler Corp. in Detroit has taken "the unprecedented step" of providing direct financial incentives to its workers enrolled in an HMO to sign up their friends. Under the plan, current members of the Health Alliance Plan of Michigan were given savings bonds of up to $250 for signing up fellow workers in the HMO.[21]

The Business Roundtable, a group made up of the chief executive officers of some 200 large U.S. companies, issued a report in February 1982 on the "appropriate role for corporations in health care cost management." Among other things, it

---

[20] "The American Health System," *op. cit.*, p. 13.
[21] See *Group Health News*, April 1983, p. 4.

recommended greater "corporate involvement in community coalitions established to address specific local health cost management problems," as well as programs to improve employee health. Many corporate executives have already discovered that it is cheaper to keep workers healthy than to pay to treat their illnesses. Thousands of companies have set up some type of physical fitness program for employees. Often these include not only exercise facilities, but also programs on nutrition, smoking, weight-control, stress management, alcohol and drug abuse, and similiar topics.[22]

Growth of Clinics; For-Profit Hospitals

An increasingly popular alternative to traditional care in hospitals and private doctors' offices is the emergency clinic, frequently set up in suburban shopping centers. It is designed to provide quick and inexpensive service for people who are willing to pay directly for the treatment of non-life-threatening emergencies. The advantages of these "emergicenters," hundreds of which have sprung up over the past few years, include immediate service, low-cost, 24-hour access, convenient location, and no need for appointments. They are not, however, a viable substitute for the hospital emergency room, where the presence of advanced support technology is required for serious emergency situations.

Despite the rise of such alternatives, the traditional, full-service hospital remains the basic structure for delivering medical care in this country. But while the number of non-profit and public hospitals has declined in recent years, the number of for-profit hospitals has rapidly increased, often by acquiring non-profit and public facilities. According to a recent article by Teresa Riordan in *The Washington Monthly,* "the for-profit hospital industry ... grew faster during the 1970s than the computer industry." [23]

Most public and non-profit hospitals were built with the help of federal funds provided through the Hill-Burton program, which required them to admit and treat charity and "bad-debt" cases as well as insured patients. But if such facilities are acquired by a for-profit chain, such as Humana Inc., Hospital Corporation of America or National Medical Enterprises, they are freed from this requirement. Critics have accused for-profit chains of favoring privately insured patients, whose policies usually reimburse the greatest amount of hospital expenses, while dumping Medicaid and non-insured patients on public

---

[22] See "Physical Fitness Boom," *E.R.R.,* 1978 Vol. I, pp. 271-273.
[23] Teresa Riordan, "The Wards Are Paved With Gold," *The Washington Monthly,* February 1983, p. 41.

and non-profit institutions. "This setup drains the already anemic philanthropic resources of publics and non-profits and often forces them to close or sell out to the for-profits," Teresa Riordan wrote.

Corporations have also taken over about half of the nation's nursing homes for the elderly. One-third of the nursing homes in this country are now owned by just 20 chains, including Beverly Enterprises and ATA Services, each of which owns 250 homes around the country. Some fear this trend may discourage the development of at-home or other community-based services for those whose conditions are not serious enough to warrant institutionalization.[24]

Providing health care for the elderly is likely to be a dominant concern for many decades. It has been estimated that the number of Americans aged 65 and older will rise steadily from the current level of 11.4 percent of the population to 21.7 percent by 2050, and that the ratio of workers to non-workers will drop from 5.4-to-1 to 2.6-to-1 over the same period.[25] This "graying of America" is expected to increase the portion of the nation's wealth allocated to health care from 10 percent today to 11 or 12 percent by the end of the century.

Ethical Issues and Budgetary Constraints

While nearly everyone agrees that more must be done to hold down increases in health care costs, some fear that cost-containment initiatives may adversely affect the quality of health care in the United States. Among those expressing this concern were the members of a presidential commission on medical ethics, whose recently released final report concluded: "Efforts to contain rising health costs are important but should not focus on limiting the attainment of equitable access for the least well served portion of the public. The achievement of equitable access is an obligation of sufficient moral urgency to warrant devoting the necessary resources to it." [26]

> The commission recognizes that efforts to rein in currently escalating health care costs have an ethical aspect because the call for adequate health care for all may not be heeded until such efforts are undertaken [the report continued]. . . . But measures

---

[24] For background, see "Housing Options for the Elderly," *E.R.R.*, 1982 Vol. II, pp. 569-588.

[25] Jerome A. Halperin, "Forces of Change in Health Services," address delivered to the College of Pharmacy, University of Arizona at Tucson, Nov. 12, 1982. Halperin is acting director of the Office of Drugs in the Food and Drug Administration.

[26] President's Commission for the Study of Ethical Problems in Medicine and Biomedical and Behavioral Research, "Securing Access to Health Care: A Report on the Ethical Implications of Differences in the Availability of Health Services," Vol. I, March 1983, pp. 5-6. Copies of the report can be obtained, at a cost of $6, from the Government Printing Office, Washington, D.C. 20402. The 11-member commission was established by Congress in 1980. Its chairman was Morris B. Abram, former president of Brandeis University.

designed to contain health care costs that exacerbate existing inequities or impede the achievement of equity are unacceptable from a moral standpoint. Moreover, they are unlikely by themselves to be successful since they will probably lead to a shifting of costs to other entities, rather than to a reduction of total expenditures.

The report did not comment on specific legislative proposals to reduce health care expenses, but it did address some of the current controversies. For example, it was critical of proposals to charge Medicaid recipients a nominal fee for each day in the hospital or each visit to a doctor's office. "Even a small out-of-pocket charge can constitute a substantial burden for some Medicaid participants," it said. The report also came out against reductions in federal funding of Medicaid, saying this "would worsen existing inequities in the distribution of the cost of care." However, the commission did express support for the idea of reducing federal tax subsidies of health insurance, as the Reagan administration has proposed *(see p. 28)*. "If properly designed, it is unlikely that such measures would compromise access to adequate health care [nor would they have] a disproportionate impact on the most economically vulnerable people. . . ," the commission stated.

Bringing medical inflation under control without jeopardizing the quality of health care in the United States will not be an easy task. But some experts see reasons for optimism. Yankelovich, Skelly and White, in their report for *Prevention* magazine, predicted that consumers will become less deferential in dealing with physicians, challenging doctors' judgments about diagnosis, treatments, costs, etc. Not only will this help control costs, the report stated, but it could change the nature of the medical profession, since physicians will be forced to become more people-oriented. At the same time, U.S. corporations are likely to continue their efforts to hold down medical costs. "In sum," the report concluded, "all of the key actors are either poised for change or will be unable to resist the pull of change. And, given the way these groups are assessing the problems and formulating strategies, there is no reason to think that either the quality of care or the equity of its distribution will diminish. They could even improve."

Selected Bibliography

Books

Davis, Karen and Cathy Schoen, *Health and the War on Poverty: A Ten-Year Appraisal,* Brookings, 1978.

Kennedy, Edward M., *In Critical Condition: The Crisis in America's Health Care,* Simon & Schuster, 1972.

Maxwell, Robert J., *Health and Wealth,* Lexington Books, 1981.

Pechman, Joseph A., ed., *Setting National Priorities: Agenda for the 1980s,* Brookings, 1980.

Pauly, Mark V., ed., *National Health Insurance: What Now, What Later, What Never?* American Enterprise Institute, 1980.

Starr, Paul, *The Social Transformation of American Medicine,* Basic Books, 1982.

Thompson, Margaret C., ed., *Health Policy: The Legislative Agenda,* Congressional Quarterly Inc., 1980.

Articles

Keisling, Phil, "Radical Surgery: Let's Draft the Doctors," *The Washington Monthly,* February 1983.

The New England Journal of Medicine, selected issues.

Seidman, Bert, "Bad Medicine for Health Care Costs," *AFL-CIO American Federationist,* April-June 1982.

Starr, Paul, "The Laissez-Faire Elixir," *The New Republic,* April 18, 1983.

"Treating the Ailing Health Care Dollar," *Journal of American Insurance,* winter 1981-82.

Reports and Studies

Congressional Budget Office, "Prospects for Medicare's Hospital Insurance Trust Fund," February 1983.

Editorial Research Reports: "Controlling Health Costs," 1977 Vol. I, p. 61; "Health Maintenance Organizations," 1974 Vol. II, p. 601; "Health Care in Britain and America," 1973 Vol. I, p. 437; "Future of Health Insurance," 1970 Vol. I, p. 61.

President's Commission for the Study of Ethical Problems in Medicine and Biomedical and Behavioral Research, "Securing Access to Health Care," March 1983.

U.S. Department of Health and Human Services, Public Health Service, "Health, United States, 1982," 1982.

Cover illustration by Staff Artist Robert Redding.

CHRONIC PAIN: THE HIDDEN EPIDEMIC

by

Marc Leepson

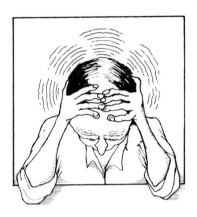

**May 27
1 9 8 3**

CHRONIC PAIN:
THE HIDDEN EPIDEMIC

MILLIONS of Americans suffer from a disease for which no medical specialty exists. This condition is scarcely taught in medical schools, and in many cases doctors are unable to diagnose, treat or relieve the problem. The disease in question is chronic pain, usually defined as any type of persistent pain that lasts more than six months. Dr. John Bonica, professor of anesthesiology at the University of Washington School of Medicine in Seattle and the founder of the nation's first chronic pain clinic, characterizes chronic pain as a "hidden epidemic." "Nearly one-third of the [U.S.] population has persistent or recurrent chronic pain," Dr. Bonica said, "and of those, one-half to two-thirds are either partially or totally disabled for periods of days, weeks or months, and sometimes permanently." [1]

Although most prevalent in older persons, chronic pain affects all age groups, and does not discriminate on the basis of sex, race or ethnic origin. Chronic pain not only causes untold physical discomfort for tens of millions of persons, it also accounts for billions of dollars in medical bills, disability payments and lost productivity and income. The total annual cost is about $50 billion, according to estimates by the National Institutes of Health (NIH). [2] The approximately 40 million Americans who suffer from chronic headaches account for $4 billion of that total (see p. 48). Migraine sufferers alone lose an estimated 65 million workdays a year due to the debilitating effects of that type of headache.

The most common form of chronic pain is backache, especially low-back pain (see p. 46). Experts believe about seven million Americans suffer from back pain so severe that they are either partially disabled or unable to work. Other common types of chronic pain are associated with cancer, arthritis and malfunctioning nerves. One of the most perplexing types of chronic pain is phantom limb pain, in which an amputee experiences extremely painful, burning sensations in what feels like the amputated limb.

[1] Quoted by Melinda Blau in "Conquering Pain: New Treatments, New Hope," *New York*, March 22, 1982, p. 27.
[2] National Institutes of Health, National Institute of Neurological and Communicative Disorders and Stroke, "Chronic Pain: Hope Through Research," April 1982, p. 2.

There are important differences between chronic pain and the "normal," everyday pain people feel when, for example, they step on a tack or twist an ankle. Doctors refer to the latter type of pain as acute pain. Acute pain may hurt, but it may also be construed as beneficial because it alerts the body to a possible injury. Although some types of chronic pain are initially triggered by a discernible factor, such as a sprained back or an infection, other types of chronic pain have no identifiable cause. This is one reason doctors have not been able to help many chronic pain sufferers. "The doctor is trained to look for a 'thorn,' " said chronic pain specialist John Liebeskind, a professor of psychology at the University of California at Los Angeles (UCLA). "But it's often the case in chronic pain that either there is no thorn, or, if it's there, it's unfindable."

Body's Reaction to Painful Sensations

Much of our understanding about how the body reacts to both acute and chronic pain has come about only in the last 15 years or so. Pain specialists readily admit that medical science does not yet completely understand how the complex system of nerves sends pain sensations to the brain. Doctors do know that the body has a separate pain system made up of countless small nerve cells whose sole job is to be acutely sensitive to physically harmful or destructive stimulation — what are called noxious stimuli. This network of cells responds to pain by sending coded electrical impulses to other cells in the brain. Some of these nerve cells are activated only by certain types of noxious stimuli; some respond both to noxious and innocuous stimuli.

Professor Liebeskind characterized the pain pathway system as a type of funnel: "At the small end — the peripheral nerves [those that supply the muscles and skin] — things are relatively clear. But as we go up and up, the system funnels out and gets more broadly distributed throughout the nervous system. It's not just a nice, thin track of 'copper wires' going from the fingers to the specialized little point in the brain that receives all messages about pain." Among the things doctors do not understand is how the various nerve cells differentiate between painful and pleasurable signals as they get distributed throughout the nervous system.

The body reacts to some types of chronic pain in a manner similar to the way it reacts to acute pain. A tumor, for example, or a swollen disc in the spinal column can press against a nerve and activate the pain pathways in the same way stepping on a tack would. Professor Liebeskind described this type of chronic pain as "a kind of acute pain that keeps happening." Other types of chronic pain, including the intense facial pain known as trigeminal neuralgia and other types of nerve pain, are caused

The Pain of Arthritis

Arthritis is a painful disease of the joints. Some 20 million Americans suffer from the various forms of arthritis; the disease accounts for more than $4 billion annually in lost income, productivity and health-care costs. There are two major types of arthritis, osteoarthritis and rheumatoid arthritis. Osteoarthritis usually affects those over 50, causing pain and redness in the fingers and sometimes in the spine and hips. Rheumatoid arthritis most often appears in people between the ages of 25 and 50. It causes inflammation, congestion and thickening of the soft tissues around the joints. Aspirin is commonly prescribed to relieve pain for most arthritis sufferers.

when the nerve pathways malfunction or are destroyed and consequently send distorted messages to the spinal cord and brain. One yet-to-be-proven theory holds that when a nerve malfunctions, some type of compensatory abnormal nerve activity takes place in the central nervous system that results in continuous (chronic) pain.

Experts believe another type of chronic pain is caused by disorders in the body's natural pain inhibitory system. Ten years ago researchers working independently in Scotland and the United States discovered that the human brain produces pain-suppressing chemical substances closely related to opiates such as morphine.[3] These substances, known as endorphins ("the morphine within"), are released by the brain and transmitted throughout the body for use in critical moments of stress and injury. When the endorphins reach the spinal cord nerve cells, they kill pain by soothing and quieting the activated nerve cells. When the body does not produce endorphins, pain continues and becomes chronic.

Although the exact causes of chronic pain are still being investigated, doctors know that psychological factors often are an important part of the problem. Dr. Lorenz Ng, a neurologist who heads the Washington (D.C.) Pain Center, described a hypothetical example: "Take the worker who injures his back on the job. Say he does not like his job. After his injury, his supervisor pays attention to him because there's compensation involved. The worker gets attention. Finally, he recovers sufficiently to go back to work. The second day on the job he bends over and the pain comes back again, as severe as before." Dr. Ng said this is not an example of malingering or faking injury, but an instance in which the pain sufferer's noxious stimuli is emotional rather than physical. "Initially injury can bring on the pain problem," Dr. Ng said. "But all you need later on is insult — the insult of the environment or the insult of the situa-

[3] See "Brain Research," *E.R.R.*, 1978 Vol. II, pp. 661-680.

tion. . . . You need to look at all factors, not just from a physical standpoint and not just from an emotional standpoint."

Still another problem doctors have in treating chronic pain is that pain cannot be measured objectively, and different persons react differently to the same amounts of pain. Doctors, therefore, must base their diagnoses primarily on what their patients tell them. "All you can really say is that if someone's degree of disability is very, very high, no matter what the pain, you have to treat it," said Dr. Godfrey Pearlson, director of the Johns Hopkins School of Medicine Pain Clinic in Baltimore.

Backaches: Most Common Pain Problem

Experts believe as many as 75 million Americans have recurring back problems. Backaches and low-back pain result in some 16 million doctor visits a year.[4] Some 200,000 Americans undergo back surgery each year. About 80 percent of those operations are unsuccessful; the patients' back pain recurs some time later. According to Steve Rothenberg, technical administrator of the Walker Pain Institute in Los Angeles, one of the most common back operations, the laminectomy,[5] "usually causes the patient to get worse because it leaves scar tissue. When it works, it works beautifully. But when it doesn't work — 80 percent of the time — it causes more pain."

One reason for the low rate of success in treating back pain is that many physicians find the problem especially difficult to deal with. "Lingering back pain is emasculating, devitalizing, fatiguing and commonly causes depression," said Dr. Bernard Jacobs, an orthopedic surgeon at the Cornell University Medical College and Hospital for Special Surgery in New York City. "It is also unusually mysterious." [6] The mystery comes from the fact that in many cases doctors are unable to find the physical cause of the pain. "Essentially, it's an invisible handicap that shows no external signs in many cases and it's very difficult to evaluate and treat," said Alan Morris, a physical therapist who is clinical director of the North Texas Back Institute in Plano, Texas. "There's a lot of room for failure and frustration. . . . Many orthopedists, neurosurgeons, neurologists and anesthesiologists . . . do not like to take care of people with back pain."

Most of those who experience back pain have relatively minor injuries in the lower back. The treatment most often prescribed is bed rest in combination with aspirin or a muscle relaxant drug such as Valium. Doctors believe a large percentage of

---

[4] Unpublished data compiled by the National Center for Health Statistics.
[5] The laminectomy involves surgical removal of a vertebra's posterior arch. In about a third of the operations, surgeons also remove a protruding disk and fuse part of the spine.
[6] Quoted in *The New York Times*, Jan. 12, 1982.

How to Prevent Backaches

Back experts say that many potential backaches can be avoided by following these suggestions:

Sitting - Millions of parents have admonished their children to "sit up straight." It turns out that this is the best way to avoid putting extra stress on the lower back while seated. The lower back should be pressed flat against the back of the chair. The feet should be flat on the floor with the knees resting at or above hip level. Crossing one leg over the other or resting one or both feet on a small stool also takes pressure off the lower back muscles. It's also important not to sit for prolonged periods.

Driving - You should also sit up straight when driving, with the small of the back pressed flat against the seatback. Make sure the seat is positioned so that you have to move only your feet and ankles — rather than the knees and hips — to work the floor pedals. During long drives it is best to stop and stretch the legs and back muscles periodically.

Standing - Those who must stand for long periods of time should try to elevate one foot four to six inches above the floor to help alleviate pressure on the back.

Sleeping - A firm mattress is best for back care while sleeping. If your mattress is very soft it can cause you to sleep with an exaggerated arch in the curve of the back. This often causes pain and stiffness. The best sleeping position is on the back or the side. Sleeping on your stomach invites back trouble because it puts extra stress on the lower back.

Lifting - Lifting heavy objects is a common cause of back pain. Those persons who have weak abdominal muscles or tensed-up back muscles also risk injury when lifting even light objects if they lift them incorrectly. The best way to lift any object is to bend the knees, keep the back straight and the stomach muscles tensed. The object should be held close to the body so that most of the pressure is on the legs and not on the back.

Source: Tufts-New England Medical Center, "What You Can Do About Back Aches," 1978.

backaches are caused by preventable factors such as obesity, weak abdominal muscles, and poor posture *(see box, above)*. During periods of stress and tension many persons involuntarily tense up their back muscles. Prolonged tension can cause those muscles to become permanently constricted. If you call upon tensed up muscles to perform — when you bend down to pick up a heavy object, work long hours in the garden, mop the floor or play softball, for example — you risk overstraining and injuring these weak muscles.

"From the backs I see, 70 or 80 percent could have been prevented if patients had kept their weight down, their back extensor muscles loose and their stomach muscles strong," said

Dr. Willibald Nagler, physiatrist-in-chief at the New York Hospital-Cornell Medical Center. Dr. Howard G. Thistle of the New York University Medical Center's Institute of Rehabilitative Medicine agreed. "We live in a push-button society, getting more and more gadgets and equipment to do things for us so that we can sit and lie down more," he said. " I think there's a whole segment of the population that has just deteriorated in terms of muscle conditioning so that they're sitting ducks for backaches." [7]

Back specialists today increasingly recommend preventive treatments for these types of backaches. The treatments often include an exercise regime to strengthen the abdominal muscles and make the back muscles flexible. Also included is advice on how to lose weight and how to sleep, sit, stand and drive without putting extra stress on the back. The YMCA, for example, has been offering a six-week "Healthy Back" program throughout the country since 1974. Treatment is much more complicated for those who suffer from chronic back pain that is not the result of weak muscles, including those with disc disease in which the back joints and discs wear out over time and are unable to support the back properly. Analysts estimate that about 2 percent of back-pain sufferers wind up with chronic pain for life.

Discomfort Caused by Chronic Headaches

Next to backaches, headaches are the most common chronic pain ailments. There are two basic types of headaches: muscular (or tension) headaches, caused by continuous contraction of the muscles in the head and neck, and vascular headaches, caused by disturbances in the flow of blood in the head. Migraine headaches are classified as vascular. Some chronic headache sufferers have both migraine and muscular headaches.

Migraine headaches are one of the most perplexing medical mysteries. Doctors do not know the cause of migraines, which last from three hours to three days and are characterized by an intense throbbing on one side of the head and usually are accompanied by nausea. What is known is that more women than men suffer from migraines. Current research is focusing on hereditary factors and dietary factors, the role of prescription drugs (such as birth control pills), "recreational" drug and alcohol use, and tension and anxiety levels. "Migraines often start in childhood and generally cease in the fifties and sixties," said Dr. David Coddon, director of the Headache Clinic at the Mount Sinai Medical Center in New York. "Migraine patients

---

[7] Drs. Nagler and Thistle were quoted by Deborah Blumenthal in "Preventing Aching Backs," *The New York Times Magazine,* Dec. 12, 1982, p. 152. A physiatrist is a physician specializing in physical rehabilitation.

usually suffer from car sickness and allergies in childhood, and they frequently have low blood pressure, low blood sugar and thyroid disturbances and menstrual irregularities." [8]

More men than women suffer from cluster headaches, a type of migraine that usually lasts from 10 minutes to three hours and recurs intermittently during the day. These headaches can be accompanied by nasal congestion. Other vascular headaches vary in frequency and intensity, and often last for three to five days. Vascular headaches, in which the pain usually is focused over the forehead or at the temples, typically begin when the person wakes up in the morning and last about three hours.

Drugs are the standard treatment for headaches. But some doctors work with headache sufferers to try to eliminate the suspected causes, including heavy drinking, irregular sleeping patterns, overeating and overmedication. Headache specialists also offer a number of relaxation techniques to overcome headache pain. These include biofeedback, progressive relaxation exercises, deep breathing and psychological counseling. Acupuncture and laser therapy have also been used with success in treating some chronic headache patients.

Growth of Pain Clinics

DR. JOHN BONICA of the University of Washington opened the first chronic pain clinic in the United States in 1960 in Seattle. Since then more than 800 clinics have been set up around the nation to treat those with chronic pain. There are two basic types of pain clinics: multi-disciplinary and unimodal. The multi-disciplinary approach, which was pioneered by Dr. Bonica, is a holistic type of treatment; the patient is examined by several specialists, ranging from neurosurgeons to psychologists, and many different types of treatments are offered. Unimodal pain clinics offer only one type of medical specialty, and typically are run by neurosurgeons or orthopedic surgeons. Other types of chronic pain clinics offer only one type of treatment, such as biofeedback therapy or acupuncture, or treat only one type of chronic pain, most often headaches or backaches.

Nearly all chronic pain sufferers first seek medical help from their family physician. Typically they are then referred to a specialist, most often a neurologist (a doctor who specializes in treating diseases of the nervous system), orthopedist (a special-

---

[8] Quoted in *U.S. News & World Report*, May 24, 1982, p. 73.

ist in skeletal problems) or neurosurgeon (a surgeon who specializes in nerve surgery). Most of those who turn to chronic pain clinics do so only after a specialist is unable to relieve their symptoms.

Multi-disciplinary clinics, most of which are affiliated with large hospitals or medical colleges, often find things other physicians have missed in trying to help chronic pain sufferers. On the other hand, these types of clinics typically do not have very high success rates because they tend to attract many "hard-core" patients — persons who have complicated health problems that have failed to respond to different types of treatments. "By the time patients get to us, they usually have not responded to conventional health care approaches," said Dr. Lorenz Ng. "They've had tests over and over again and nothing seems to explain the pain."

This is one reason the multi-disciplinary clinics offer many different types of specialists. The Pain Clinic at Johns Hopkins University School of Medicine, for example, is staffed by an array of physicians and therapists, including psychiatrists, neurologists, neurosurgeons and occupational and physical therapists. "One of the hospital's chaplains even has an active interest in it," said the clinic's director, Dr. Godfrey Pearlson. At the Walker Pain Institute in Los Angeles, a private clinic that handles some 15,000 patient visits a year, the specialists and therapists are trained by Dr. Judith Walker, a neurophysiologist and anesthesiologist who has developed a number of treatment techniques. The three-year-old center also is involved in chronic pain research.

The Washington (D.C.) Pain Center run by Dr. Ng, who formerly headed the pain studies program at the National Institute of Drug Abuse, uses a "systems" approach in treating patients. "We take a look at the whole system and the importance of one level that impinges upon the other," Dr. Ng said. "Treatment needs to be coordinated. You need to look at the physical as well as the psycho-social, the environmental and the emotional aspects." The center's staff includes clinical psychologists, physical therapists and a biofeedback specialist. The treatments offered include various types of electrical nerve stimulation *(see p. 57)* as well as therapeutic sessions to help patients deal with stress, and assertiveness training classes.

Lack of Training in U.S. Medical Schools

One reason for the proliferation of clinics is that it is difficult to find an individual physician skilled in diagnosing and treating chronic pain. This is because most American medical schools do not provide students with the training needed to work with chronic pain sufferers. "Fifty to 60 million people a year suffer from chronic pain, yet medical schools right now devote probably one or two pages in a textbook . . . to treatment of chronic pain," said Steve Rothenberg of the Walker Pain Institute. "We have the necessary tools to treat this kind of pain successfully, but most physicians in the United States are unaware of them and are sorely lacking in education. It's not necessarily their own fault, but the fact is that the whole system right now isn't set up for chronic pain."

Some medical schools and pain clinics are working to remedy that situation. At Johns Hopkins School of Medicine, for example, a recently instituted program rotates many residents through the school's pain clinic. Neurosurgery and psychiatry residents typically spend several months helping treat chronic pain patients in the clinic. The university also offers lectures on chronic pain to first-year medical students. Private clinics, such as the Walker Pain Institute, also have begun training residents. The Walker clinic has a program in which UCLA medical students observe the institute's operations and learn the various chronic pain treatments offered there.

It's clear, though, that chronic pain clinics will continue to offer more hope for pain patients than will individual physicians. One reason is that many doctors in private practice do not have the facilities to treat the different types of chronic pain. "Many physicians don't have the support personnel to help them," said Alan Morris of the North Texas Back Institute. "It's not like taking out an appendix where you go in and do the surgery and you're out. Very often [chronic pain patients] have long, ongoing problems. There are frequently psychological considerations. . . . Dealing with that takes some supportive personnel."

Some Specialized Pain Treatment Clinics

Studies indicate that 50-60 percent of terminal cancer patients suffer from chronic pain, some of it related to such cancer treatments as radiology and chemotherapy. The Pain Clinic at Memorial Sloan-Kettering Cancer Center in New York City specializes in treating pain in cancer patients. The clinic, under the direction of neurologist Dr. Kathleen Foley, also is involved in chronic pain research to find out how pain is related to the underlying cancer. "In contrast to other pain clinics where people spend a lot of time just treating pain, we treat cancer — the cause of the pain — as well," Dr. Foley said in an interview.

The clinic offers different types of pain treatments, but most patients are given drugs to relieve their pain. The type of drug and the dosage depend on a series of factors. "It depends on the age of the patients, their prior narcotic exposure and the degree of pain," Dr. Foley said. "If you have a patient with mild pain, you might give them aspirin. If you have a patient with severe acute pain you give them intramuscular morphine." Most often the clinic comes up with a combination of drugs for each patient. The objective is to find a drug combination that relieves the pain, has few side effects and keeps the patient alert and attentive.

It was once thought that a combination of drugs and alcohol called Bromptom's mix was the answer to that problem. The mixture was invented by British physician Cicely Saunders, the developer of the modern-day hospice, the non-hospital treatment center for terminal cancer patients.[9] The concoction was made up of powerful drugs such as heroin or morphine, alcohol and a sugar syrup. But after the effects of the mix had been closely studied for several years, it was found that the various ingredients did not work to relieve pain any more effectively than morphine alone. British and American hospices now usually give terminal patients oral morphine, which dulls pain and keeps them alert.

Several pain clinics across the nation specialize in treating longtime headache sufferers. The Diamond Headache Clinic, which is associated with the Chicago Medical School Department of Neurology, sees about 2,000 new patients a year and handles some 14,000 follow-up visits annually. Each new patient undergoes a complete physical and neurological examination that includes blood tests, skull X-rays and brain wave monitoring. The patient's medical history, including family history of headaches and other disorders, is checked. Patients are asked to describe the location of their headaches, their frequency, severity, associated symptoms and how the pain affects sleeping patterns. Female migraine sufferers are asked to keep track of the relationship between their migraines and their menstrual cycles. Patients also are asked to keep a diary to record the severity of their headaches and the effect of their medication. After the diagnosis is completed, an individualized treatment program is devised. Most often it involves analgesic drugs or biofeedback (see p. 58)

Dozens of clinics specializing in helping patients with chronic back pain have been set up across the nation in recent years. The North Texas Back Institute near Dallas, for example, opened its doors in 1979. Its patients include those who have been hospitalized for back and spinal problems as well as those with relatively minor back problems. All are referred to the clinic by physicians. The institute's philosophy is to get patients

---

[9] See "The Hospice Movement," *E.R.R.*, 1980 Vol. II, pp. 821-840.

Where to Find Relief

Some of the nation's top chronic pain clinics include:

Diamond Headache Clinic
The Chicago Medical School
Department of Neurology
Chicago, Ill. 60625
312-878-5558

Emory University Pain
  Control Center
Center for Rehabilitation
  Medicine
1441 Clifton Rd, N.E.
Atlanta, Ga. 30322
404-329-5492

Johns Hopkins University
  School of Medicine
Pain Clinic
600 N. Wolfe St.
Baltimore, Md. 21205
301-955-3270

Massachusetts Rehabilita-
  tion Hospital
Boston Pain Unit
Boston, Mass. 02114
617-720-6510

Mayo Clinic
Pain Center
200 First St. S.W.
Rochester, Minn. 55905
507-284-8311

Memorial Sloan-Kettering
  Cancer Center
Pain Clinic
1275 York Ave
New York, N.Y. 10021
212-794-7050

Mount Sinai Medical Center
Pain Center
Miami Beach, Fla. 33140
305-674-2070

Mount Sinai Medical
  Center
Headache Clinic
1 Gustave Levy Place
New York, N.Y. 10019
212-650-7691

Nebraska Pain Rehabilita-
  tion Unit
42nd and Dewey
Omaha, Neb. 68105
402-559-4364

New Hope Pain Center and
  Pain Research Foundation
Alhambra Community
  Hospital
100 S. Raymond Ave.
Alhambra, Calif. 91801
213-570-1607

New York University
  Medical Center
Pain Consultation Service
530 First Ave.
New York, N.Y. 10020
212-340-7316

North Texas Back Institute
3801 W. 15th St.
Plano, Texas 75075
214-867-2720

Northwest Pain Center
  Associates
10615 S.E. Cherry Blossom
  Dr.
Portland, Ore. 97216
503-256-1930

Rehabilitation Institute of
  Chicago
Center for Pain Studies
345 E. Superior St.
Chicago, Ill. 60611
312-649-6011

UCLA Pain Management
  Center
10833 Le Conte Ave.
Los Angeles, Calif. 90024
213-825-4292

University of Washington
  School of Medicine
Pain Clinic
1959 N.E. Pacific St.
Seattle, Wash. 98195
206-543-3236

involved in their own preventive treatments. "We believe that most of what people feel as back pain is related to the number of things they do over time that accumulate and accelerate the degenerative or wearing-out process," said Alan Morris, the institute's clinical director. "We try to help the patients understand a little bit about the anatomical structure involved to help them understand how the things they do every day affect that wearing-out process. Once they understand that, they can apply some of the simple behavioral and postural changes that will help them allow their spines to rest more effectively and to slow down that degenerative process."

Widespread Use of Pain-Relieving Drugs

Despite the plethora of treatments available at chronic pain clinics, drugs remain the most prescribed treatment for the ailment. Among the drugs, aspirin is one of the most frequently used. Medical science does not know precisely how aspirin works; nevertheless, it provides relief for many headache, backache and arthritis sufferers. "Scientists still cannot explain all the ways aspirin works," an NIH publication said, "but they do know that it interferes with pain signals where they usually originate, at the ... nerve endings outside the brain and the spinal cord: peripheral nerves." [10] Aspirin is not addictive, but it does have side effects in some persons. Some are allergic to it; in others it irritates the lining of the stomach. An alternative for those who cannot take aspirin is a drug called acetaminophen, sold under trade names such as Tylenol. That substance does not irritate the stomach, but sometimes is not effective in relieving pain.

In cases where aspirin or acetaminophen are not strong enough, doctors often recommend powerful prescription drugs, such as codeine, Darvon, morphine, Demerol, Inderal, Motrin and Indocin. But these drugs often bring unwanted side effects and can be dangerous when taken in combination with other drugs or alcohol.[11] Sometimes a pain patient can become psychologically dependent on the drugs, although research indicates that most chronic pain sufferers who use strong drugs do not become addicted. "Cancer patients who take a lot of drugs for a period of time [usually] can just stop taking them," said Dr. Foley of the Sloan-Kettering Pain Clinic.

Nevertheless, some chronic pain patients do become psychologically dependent on the drugs they use to fight pain. Buddy Dial, a former star football player with the Pittsburgh Steelers and Dallas Cowboys, for example, used Darvon, Percodan,

---

[10] National Institutes of Health, *op. cit.*, p. 14.
[11] See "Prescription-Drug Abuse," *E.R.R.*, 1982 Vol. I, pp. 429-448.

Demerol and Pergonal after a series of back operations. Dial's drug addiction caused him to lose interest in life. His business folded; his wife divorced him. He wound up living as an invalid in his parents' house. "I completely withdrew," Dial said. "I'd wake up, take a shot or pill and then go back to sleep. . . . I don't know how many times Mother and Daddy had to rush me to the hospital when I'd go into convulsions from taking too much." [12] Dial overcame his addiction with the help of some former teammates who took him to a pain clinic where he was weaned off drugs. He instead began using non-drug treatments including self-hypnosis and stretching exercises.

Another public figure who has overcome addiction to pain-killing drugs is former first lady Betty Ford. In 1978 Mrs. Ford voluntarily entered Long Beach Naval Hospital for 28 days of treatment for alcohol and drug dependence. Mrs. Ford, whose main problem was alcoholism, began taking pain-killing drugs while recovering from a mastectomy. Today Mrs. Ford is cured of her alcoholism and drug dependency, and works with drug and alcohol rehabilitation programs. She gives weekly lectures at a new $5-million, 60-bed alcoholic treatment center in Rancho Mirage, Calif.

Advances in Treatments

IN THE LAST DECADE medical science has made significant breakthroughs in learning about the workings of the nervous system and the brain. This research has led to the development of many innovative types of pain treatment techniques. Additionally, researchers are working on dozens of promising new projects that, added to the body of existing knowledge, promise to give physicians a continually growing arsenal of pain-relieving techniques. "We are much more sophisticated about the nature of pain and the methods of relieving it than we were even five years ago," said Dr. Kathleen Foley. "And we have learned more about pain in the last 10 years than in the previous one hundred." [13]

Today's physicians have the unique advantage of being able to use advanced technological treatments as well as age-old pain relief methods. One of the oldest is acupuncture, the traditional Chinese medical treatment. Acupuncture has been used as a general anesthetic for thousands of years in medical procedures

[12] Writing in *People*, Jan. 17, 1983, p. 36.
[13] Quoted by Ellen Switzer, "Pain," *Vogue,* May 1981, p. 313

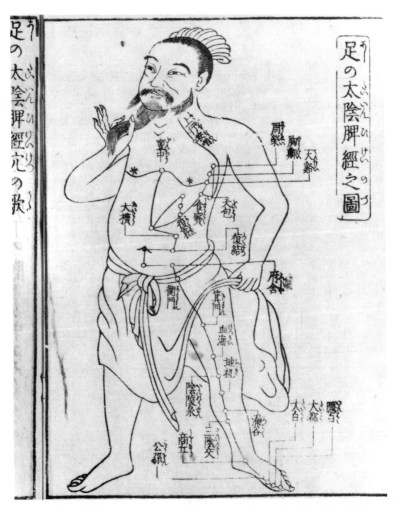

Acupuncture points are indicated in this Japanese version of the traditional Chinese medical treatment.

ranging from pulling teeth to childbirth. To ease chronic pain the acupuncturist inserts a series of very fine metal needles into the skin at several of the 800 acupuncture points in the body that run along 14 lines, or meridians. It is not known precisely how acupuncture works, but research indicates that the needles somehow stimulate or repress the functions of the nervous system.

Western interest in acupuncture grew following President Nixon's 1972 trip to China. Since then, many acupuncture specialists have set up shop in this country and chronic pain patients have been treated successfully with the technique. Nevertheless, the jury is still out on acupuncture's effectiveness in alleviating most types of chronic pain. According to the National Institutes of Health: "Current opinion is that more controlled trials are needed to define which pain conditions might be helped by acupuncture and which patients are most likely to benefit." [14]

New Types of Electric Nerve Stimulation

There are several treatment techniques that involve electrical stimulation of the nerves. These techniques, which apply brief jolts of electricity to nerve endings, evolved from ancient treatments using electric eels to shock patients out of their pain. The most common treatment today is transcutaneous ("through the skin") electrical nerve stimulation, known as TENS or TNS. The technique, which has been called a type of "electrical aspirin," involves applying brief pulses of electricity to nerve endings under the skin. The electricity comes from a small battery-powered impulse generator known as a stimulator. The electricity reaches the body through electrodes attached to the skin. As is the case with acupuncture, the electrodes are not necessarily hooked onto the area of pain; sometimes the electrodes are attached at the same points acupuncturists use.

The exact reason why this technique works to relieve pain still remains a mystery. Researchers theorize that the electrical current somehow blocks the nerves from sending pain signals to the brain or that the current activates the release of endorphins from the brain *(see p. 45)*. Success rates vary from 25-80 percent, depending on the type of pain. Patients can rent or purchase portable TENS generators, and the treatment is covered by many health insurance policies. A similar technique, subcutaneous ("under the skin") nerve stimulation (SCNS), electronically stimulates the nerves underneath the skin. SCNS was developed by Dr. Judith Walker of the Walker Pain Institute in Los Angeles, and has been used successfully to treat patients with chronic pelvic pain and certain types of back pain and neuralgia.

Experiments are now taking place with the ultimate electrical nerve stimulation technique, neural stimulation, in which electric current is applied directly to the brain. What could be the most promising type of nerve stimulation, using low-power laser beams, also is in the experimental stage.[15] Laser therapy has been used succesfully in experiments to relieve migraine, back and arthritis pain. "It takes repetitive treatments, but it seems to work quite well," said Steve Rothenberg of the Walker Pain Institute. "It doesn't stimulate like electricity stimulates or like heat stimulates. It has some kind of neurochemical effect on the

---

[14] National Institutes of Health, *op. cit.,* p. 10.
[15] For information on other medical uses of lasers, see "Lasers' Promising Future," *E.R.R.,* 1983 Vol. I, pp. 373-392.

nerves.... We think it's going to be the technology of the nineties."

Success With Hypnosis and Biofeedback

For those susceptible to its powers, hypnosis can be effective in helping block out pain. "Hypnosis is more of a science now that we've introduced the concept of first measuring a person's trance capacity and then tailoring treatment strategy accordingly," said Dr. Herbert Spiegel, a New York psychiatrist and an expert on medical uses of hypnosis.[16] Still, hypnosis is by no means universally accepted as a chronic pain treatment. An NIH report characterized its effectivness as "uncertain" because studies have shown that only about 15-20 percent of chronic pain patients get "total relief" with hypnosis. At the same time NIH recognized that hypnosis can reduce anxiety and depression for pain patients. "By lowering the burden of emotional suffering, pain may become more bearable," the report said.[17]

Biofeedback, the technique in which information about bodily functions is fed back to a patient through machines that measure minute bodily changes, has been effective in lessening the frequency and severity of chronic headaches, including migraines, and other types of pain caused by muscular tension. Some chronic headache patients have been able to stop using medication after learning relaxation techniques through biofeedback therapy. Biofeedback machines translate bodily changes such as muscular tension and temperature into information — usually variable audio tones. A patient can therefore "hear" the changes in his or her body. A biofeedback therapist working with someone suffering from chronic tension headaches, for example, attaches electrodes from an electromyograph (EMG) to the patient's forehead. The machine measures the tension in the scalp and neck muscles that causes tension headaches. The therapist teaches the patient to use relaxation techniques to release the tension and relieve the pain. As the muscles relax, the EMG's tone slows down; when the muscles tense, the machine's tone increases. The goal in biofeedback therapy is for a patient to use the relaxation techniques without the biofeedback equipment.

Other Sources of Relief from Chronic Pain

When drugs, acupuncture, electronic nerve stimulation and other pain treatments fail, some physicians recommend a surgical technique to sever the nerves in the spinal cord or brain responsible for the pain. But this very risky procedure has some dangerous potential complications, and is only undertaken

[16] Quoted by Melinda Blau, *op. cit.,* p. 31.
[17] National Institutes of Health, *op. cit.,* p. 18.

when all other measures fail. "Surgery can bring about instant, magical release from pain," NIH reported, "but surgery may also destroy other sensations as well, or, inadvertently, become the source of new pain. Further, relief is not necessarily permanent. After six months or a year, pain may return." [18] Doctors sometimes recommend a less risky procedure, the nerve block. In this procedure an anesthetic or other substance is injected into the painful area to anesthetize the nerves responsible for the pain. Nerve blocks are temporary, however; the effects last for only about three months.

Millions of Americans seek relief from chronic pain from chiropractors. Chiropractors believe that all disease results from disruptions in the workings of the nerves that are caused primarily by the displacement of the vertebrae and the spine. Chiropractors typically treat chronic pain patients by adjusting the displaced vertebrae to try to relieve pressure on spinal nerves. The adjustments are made using a special hand massage technique. Chiropractors use other chronic pain treatments, including TENS, and applications of heat, cold, light and ultrasound (high-frequency sound used primarily to reduce spasms). Although the medical community tends to frown on chiropractic theories and treatments, the techniques have helped many chronic pain patients. Some pain specialists even recommend chiropractic therapy for certain patients.

Many multi-disciplinary pain clinics recommend exercise as a treatment for pain patients, especially those with chronic back pain. Many doctors believe that the proper type of exercise program can eliminate a large percentage of backaches. The University of Miami's Comprehensive Pain Center, for example, runs an extensive exercise program for patients who have had back surgery and for those who have been recommended for surgery. The center's staff of 50 doctors and therapists administers the program to patients for up to 12 hours a day, without bed rest. The program includes back calisthenics and even aerobic dancing. Other types of pain treatments — including the Alexander Technique (a series of movements designed to relieve stress and pain), the Feldenkrais Method (a body manipulation and exercise regimen) and various forms of deep muscle massage and pressure point therapy — involve manipulation of the muscles, and have helped relieve chronic pain in some people. But despite all the treatment options now available, even the most optimistic specialists admit that much more research needs to be done before the majority of chronic pain patients can find total relief.

---

[18] *Ibid.*, p. 20.

Selected Bibliography

Books

Benjamin, Ben E., *Listen to Your Pain,* Viking Press, 1983.
Diamond, Seymour, *The Practicing Physician's Approach to Headache,* Williams & Wilkins, 1982.
Evans, David P., *Backache: Its Evolution and Conservative Treatment,* University Park Press, 1982.
Kerr, Frederick W., *The Pain Book,* Prentice-Hall, 1981.
Kotarba, Joseph A., *Chronic Pain,* Sage Publications, 1983.
Melleby, Alexander, *The Y's Way to a Healthy Back,* New Century, 1982.
Murphy, Wendy B., *Dealing With Headaches,* Time-Life Books, 1982.
Smoller, Bruce, *Pain Control,* Doubleday, 1982.
Tollison, C. David, *Managing Chronic Pain,* Sterling, 1982.
White, Arthur H., *Back School and Other Conservative Approaches to Low Back Pain,* Mosby, 1983.

Articles

Blau, Melinda, "Conquering Pain: New Treatments, New Hope," *New York,* March 22, 1982.
Blumenthal, Deborah, "Preventing Aching Backs," *The New York Times Magazine,* Dec. 12, 1982.
"Headache Sufferers: Help is on the Way," *U.S. News & World Report,* May 24, 1982.
Johnson, Roger S., "Treating Pain in the Already Addicted Patient," *Aches & Pains,* October 1982.
Kornfeld, Joe, "Getting Aggressive About Conservative Therapy for Back Pain," *Medical World News,* July 5, 1982.
Shelton, Linda K., "Relief from Chronic Pain: Alternative Treatments," *Ms.,* January 1983.
"TENS: The Latest Way to Stop Pain," *Changing Times,* January 1982.

Reports and Studies

Belkin, Stuart C. and Henry H. Banks, "What You Can Do About Back Aches," Tufts-New England Medical Center, 1978.
Editorial Research Reports: "The Hospice Movement," 1980 Vol. II, p. 821; "Brain Research," 1978 Vol. II, p. 661.
National Institute on Drug Abuse, "New Approaches to Treatment of Chronic Pain," May 1981.
National Institutes of Health, National Institute of Neurological and Communicative Disorders and Stroke, "Chronic Pain: Hope Through Research," April 1982.

Graphics: Cover illustration by Art Director Richard Pottern; illustration p. 56 courtesy of the National Library of Medicine.

WEIGHT CONTROL: A NATIONAL OBSESSION

by

Jean Rosenblatt
and Sandra Stencel

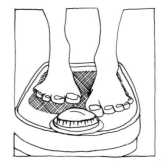

Nov. 19
1 9 8 2

Editor's Note: New height and weight tables published by the Metropolitan Life Insurance Co. on March 1, 1983, indicated that people can weigh more than they did in 1959, when the last charts were published, and still expect favorable longevity. A spokesman for the company stressed that the new weights, although higher, were still well below the weights of most Americans.

WEIGHT CONTROL:
A NATIONAL OBSESSION

FOR MOST Americans, Thanksgiving is a time for celebration, a day to spend with family and friends. It is also an excuse to stuff ourselves with turkey, sweet potatoes, pumpkin pie and other traditional treats. Nothing is wrong, of course, with occasional holiday binging. But for many, overeating is a daily temptation.

The number of Americans who are overweight is largely a matter of conjecture, since experts disagree on how fat is too fat. One set of standards that has gained wide acceptance for correlating weight with height, sex and age was devised by Metropolitan Life Insurance Co. Using this guideline, 46 percent of adult Americans are at least 10 percent overweight. According to another source, 15 percent of adult men and 25 percent of adult women are 20 percent or more overweight.[1]

Few overweight people are happy with the situation. Americans spend over $10 billion a year trying to lose weight and keep it off. At any given moment an estimated 20 million persons are thought to be on a "serious" diet. For years best-seller lists have been dominated by books by the latest diet and exercise gurus. Not surprisingly, when *The San Francisco Chronicle* asked 500 people what they feared most, 190 of them said "getting fat." [2]

While losing weight may be a national obsession, many apparently are losing the battle of the bulge. At least 95 percent of dieters gain back all the weight they have lost. "If 'cure' from obesity is defined as reduction to ideal weight and maintenance of that weight for five years, a person is more likely to recover from most forms of cancer than from obesity," wrote Kelly D. Brownell, associate professor of psychiatry at the University of Pennsylvania.[3]

While weight-conscious Americans are debating the merits of the latest fad diets, medical researchers are involved in their own debate over how much control a person has over his or her weight. Much of the controversy centers on a theory discussed

---

[1] Theodore B. Van Itallie and John G. Kral, "The Dilemma of Morbid Obesity," *Journal of the American Medical Association*, Aug. 28, 1981.
[2] *The San Francisco Chronicle*, Jan. 17, 1981.
[3] Kelly D. Brownell, "Obesity: Understanding and Treating a Serious, Prevalent, and Refractory Disorder," *Journal of Consulting and Clinical Psychology*, vol. 5, no. 6, 1982, p. 820.

in a new book by Dr. William Bennett and Joel Gurin.[4] They contend that each person has a natural "setpoint" that encourages the body to maintain a certain weight much like a thermostat keeps a room at a particular temperature *(see p. 67).* "The difference [between fat and thin people] is not between the weak and the strong or the impulsive and the abstemious, but between internal (quite probably innate) controls that are set differently in different people," they wrote in *The Dieters Dilemma: Eating Less and Weighing More* (1982).

Link Between Excess Weight, Longevity

A commonly accepted definition of obesity is "an increase in body weight beyond the limitation of skeletal and physical requirement, as the result of an excessive accumulation of fat." [5] But there is little agreement about where overweight ends and obesity begins. There is also disagreement over the health risks associated with being overweight. Studies have linked obesity to high blood pressure, gall bladder disease, arthritis, diabetes and heart disease, the nation's leading cause of death. But still unclear is the exact relationship between excess weight and longevity.[6]

Insurance industry studies, government surveys and independent research by doctors have tended to confirm the suspicion that heavyweights die young. But critics of these studies contend that they are based on information drawn from death certificates, which may not reflect underlying causes, or in some cases may be inaccurate. Dr. Reubin Andres, clinical director of the Gerontology Research Center of the National Institute on Aging in Baltimore, Md., reanalyzed data from several prominent studies and found no relationship between obesity and mortality in people less than 30 percent overweight.[7]

Bennett and Gurin point out that in the past 15 years the average male has gained four or five pounds and women slightly less. "If fat is as deadly as we have been led to believe, somebody out there should have been digging an ever-increasing number of extra-wide graves," they wrote. "But, since 1965, Americans' life expectancy has increased by a couple of years." [8]

Frequently cited as evidence that obesity contributes to a number of fatal diseases is the "Framingham study," formally the National Heart Institute's Heart Disease Epidemiology

---

[4] Bennett is associate editor of the *Harvard Medical School Health Letter* and Gurin is editor of *American Health.*
[5] Cited by Sandra Edwards in *Too Much is Not Enough* (1981), p. 50.
[6] See "Obesity and Health," *E.R.R.,* 1977 Vol. I, pp. 453-472.
[7] Reubin Andres, "Effect of Obesity on Total Mortality," *International Journal of Obesity,* vol. 4, 1980.
[8] William Bennet and Joel Gurin, *The Dieter's Dilemma* (1982), p. 109.

Study. In the late 1940s, 5,209 people living in the Boston suburb of Framingham, Mass., agreed to participate in a series of questionnaires and examinations every two years. All deaths were recorded and their causes established. The study was intended primarily to explore the causes of heart disease and stroke.

The findings of the latest Framingham study were disclosed earlier this year. After analyzing 26 years of follow-up data on the original participants, the researchers concluded that obesity, independent of its association with high blood pressure and serum cholesterol, increases a person's risk of developing cardiovascular disease. According to Dr. Helen B. Hubert, who reported the results of the study to an American Heart Association conference in San Antonio last spring, "Any increase in weight after early adulthood increases a person's risk of cardiovascular disease." [9]

Given the results of the study, Dr. Hunter is concerned about reports that Metropolitan Life Insurance Co. is revising its standards of what constitutes normal weight. The new charts are scheduled to be published early next year and, according to Frederic Seltzer, head of Metropolitan's statistical bureau, they will probably increase desirable weights by about 10 percent. Dr. Hunter believes it is premature to suggest that people can be safely heavier than now thought. "The long-term consequences could be devastating," she said.

Others would like to do away with the notion that there are ideal weights. "There are several definitions of 'desirable' weight for any one person," said Dr. Andres. "The esthetic desirable promoted by sexual competition, the media, and fashion; the life-expectancy desirable; the disease-defense desirable — all are different." [10] While a weight gain of five or 10 pounds may be damaging to a person's ego, experts agree that it is not life-threatening.

Physiological Factors in Weight Control

People gain weight when they consume more calories than their bodies burn off. But no one knows exactly why people eat to excess. According to most experts, there is no one underlying cause for obesity. "Obesity overall is a predicament of Americans, brought about by a particular social and physical environment," said Dr. Theodore Van Itallie, director of the obesity

---

[9] Quoted in *Medical World News,* April 26, 1982, p. 68. A study published by three Framingham researchers in 1980 received a lot of public attention for its conclusion that underweight persons, as well as those who are overweight, tend to have higher-than-average mortality rates. See Paul Sorlie, Tavia Gordon, and William B. Kannel, "Body Build and Mortality: The Framingham Study," *Journal of the American Medical Association,* May 9, 1980, pp. 1828-1831.

[10] Quoted by Karen Anderegg in "Are We Fatness Crazy?" *Vogue,* March 1982, p. 399.

research center at St. Luke's Hospital in New York City. "It's a byproduct of a culture that emphasizes a variety of nutritious, palatable, calorically rich foods readily available to everyone, together with a degree of mechanization that makes it very difficult to expend more than a sedentary level of energy. This combination would produce obesity in almost any species of mammal. But some humans are more responsive to this environmental situation than others." [11]

Psychological factors undoubtedly play a role in weight gain, though there is no one psychological profile of a fat person. Some people eat for neurotic reasons, to assuage anxiety or suppress anger, sadness or even happiness. Dr. Brownell believes that people can become psychologically addicted to either certain foods or to the symbolic importance of eating or overeating at certain times. The use of food to alleviate anxiety is probably determined in childhood. "People learn a number of ways to respond to emotional situations," Brownell said in a recent interview, "and we're likely to carry those over into our adult life."

In recent years experts have paid increased attention to the physiological factors involved in weight control. According to Dr. Van Itallie, a normal-weight person usually has between 30-40 billion fat cells, whereas some obese people may have between 80-120 billion. Researchers have also found that while the number of fat cells can increase, they cannot decrease, which may mean that weight gain irreversibly increases their number. Fat cell size may be another variable that helps determine body weight. Dr. Brownell speculated, "Fat cell size may set the biological limit to weight loss, whereas fat cell number may determine the weight at which this limit occurs." [12]

Researchers believe that obese people may be more sensitive to external food cues, such as the smell and sight of food, and less responsive to internal hunger cues than non-obese people, causing them to eat beyond the point of satiety. They may also be hungrier than normal-weight people. Autopsies of some overweight people have revealed damaged hypothalamuses, the area of the brain that controls hunger, sexual response, regulation of body temperature and the need for sleep. It could be that the obese receive incorrect signals concerning how full or how hungry they are, which results in an ongoing desire to eat.

Scientists have recently found a group of sites in the brain that seem to help control appetite and may dictate whether people become fat or thin. This discovery supports the idea that

[11] Interview with *Psychology Today*, October 1978.
[12] Brownell, *op. cit.*, p. 823.

Lose Fat, Not Weight

Compulsive weight watchers are apt to confuse weight with fat. Weight is not a true indication of how fat a person is because weight includes muscle and bone as well as fat. And because muscle is denser than fat, a muscular person is leaner than a fat person of the same weight. The ideal amount of body fat is about 12 percent of total weight for men and 18-20 percent for women.

People who go on low-carbohydrate or other crash diets may lose weight but not much fat. When the body is deprived of its usual energy source, it converts body protein into energy. According to a report in the March 1982 issue of the *FDA Consumer,* "this protein is taken from lean body mass muscle and major organs such as the liver, heart and kidneys." William Bennett and Joel Gurin, authors of *The Dieter's Dilemma* (1982), contend that "more than a third of the weight lost through dieting alone — and some two-thirds of the weight lost on a total fast — can reflect loss of muscle, not fat."

in some people, at least, fatness is not controlled by the amount of food they eat but by factors beyond their control — in this case, chemicals in the brain. The newly discovered areas in the brain that affect appetite are called "appetite receptors," and they have been found mainly in the hypothalamus and brain stem.[13] According to research done on laboratory mice, a genetically fat animal has more appetite receptor sites than thinner mice in the same litter, and the more sites, the greater the appetite.

"There are probably a lot of things that control appetite," said Dr. Phil Skolnick, one of the National Institutes of Health researchers involved in the project. "One thing that is possible is that there is some basic substance that we have not yet found that controls appetite through these sites. Or these sites may be the sites for the release of some neurotransmitters [brain chemicals that transmit signals between brain cells]." [14] Identification of these appetite receptor sites, which was reported in the October 1982 issue of *Science* magazine,[15] could lead to the development of an appetite-suppressing drug without undesirable side effects. And, according to *Science* reporter Gina Kolata, "it also may explain how amphetamines work and may lead to a coherent theory of how appetite is regulated." [16]

Authors William Bennett and Joel Gurin also believe that physiological rather than psychological factors dictate eating patterns. "Forces beyond conscious awareness" regulate how

[13] The brain stem is the top part of the spinal cord and the lower part of the brain. The hypothalamus is located above the brain stem.
[14] Quoted in *The Washington Post,* Oct. 23, 1982.
[15] Steven M. Paul, Bridget Hulihan-Giblin and Phil Skolnick, "Amphetamine Binding to Rat Hypothalamus," *Science,* October 1982, pp. 487-489.
[16] Gina Kolata, "Brain Receptors for Appetite Discovered," *Science,* October 1982, p. 460.

much a person eats, they wrote. "But the forces in question are not the familiar denizens of the Freudian unconscious — repressed conflict, displaced anger, infantile deprivation. They are, instead, physiological pressures to keep a foreordained amount of fat on the body." [17]

Dieting is doomed to fail, Bennett and Gurin argue, because the body will naturally balance caloric intake, metabolic efficiency and physical activity to maintain this level of stored fat, which they call the setpoint. "Your metabolic rate and your hunger change depending on whether you're below or above the setpoint," Gurin told Editorial Research Reports. "When you diet — force yourself below the setpoint — you will become hungry, obsessed by food, which is one way your body tries to get you to your setpoint. At the same time your metabolic rate will slow down as a way of conserving calories, as a defense against caloric restriction." The best way to permanently lose weight, Bennett and Gurin argue, is to lower the body's setpoint through physical exercise *(see box, p. 75)*.

Dieting as a Variable in Gaining Weight

Dieting may not only be a futile attempt to overwhelm the body's setpoint, but may actually make it harder to lose weight and easier to gain it. This assumption is based partly on growing evidence that there is nothing abnormal about the way fat people eat: they do not necessarily eat faster, snack more often or eat any more than some thinner people. What fat people do more than normal-weight people is diet.

A person who significantly reduces calorie intake may trigger the body's starvation reflex. Starvation lowers the body's metabolic rate so fewer calories are used to keep basic processes going. As a result of these adaptive changes in body metabolism, the dieter may reach a frustrating plateau during which little or no weight is lost. Metabolic changes can also create problems for successful dieters, for as soon as they resume "normal" eating they often incur a rapid weight gain.

Among those who believe that frequent dieting may be a crucial factor in weight gain are Susan and Wayne Wooley, who operate the Clinic for Eating Disorders at the University of Cincinnati College of Medicine. To support their theory they cite the following evidence:

Non-dieters whose overeating is not preceded by a period of caloric reduction gain very little weight.

People who begin eating normally after losing weight gain weight very easily, and the regained weight is mostly fat.

Obese people gain weight much more easily than non-obese people.

---

[17] Bennett and Gurin, *op. cit.*, p. 23.

Obese people almost always have a long history of dieting.[18]

"The data for our theory are not yet so strong," Susan Wooley conceded. "But if it is true, it would mean that we are doing things so much the wrong way.... We should be taking a very close look at all the aspects of metabolism after dieting."[19]

Standards of Beauty

FAT people suffer untold humiliation in a society that reveres thinness and sees fat as deviant and repulsive. A common attitude is that expressed by a formerly fat journalist: "If I could lose weight so can they. Their fat just shows that they're gluttons. There's no excuse." Doctors, employers, college admissions personnel and salespeople have all been said to discriminate against fat people, whose psychological problems may be more a result of their fatness than the cause of it.

"If excess weight were the problem, clearly losing it would be the solution," Susan Edwards wrote in *Too Much is Not Enough* (1981). "Instead overweight is often the byproduct of what started out as an assuagement, overeating. In tempering emotional or biochemical responses with food, the original fears, frustrations, and maladjustments became transmuted, and fat, the result of the solution, becomes the problem itself. Now all blame for fears and frustrations can be ascribed to fat, and all hope invested in another external change, its loss."

According to psychologist Susan Wooley, obese people may hide from the world and forgo a normal life until they lose weight, believing that thinness will end all personal difficulties. But even if fat people lose weight they often remain unhappy. "I felt intense disappointment after a large weight loss," said one woman. "My heart was broken when my fantasies about thinness ... ran into the reality of thinness. All was *not* well.... I was lonely and depressed and right up against the very emptiness I had always eaten over."[20]

Desperation dieting in some cases can lead to a severe loss of weight. The saddest and most extreme examples are people suffering from a psychological disorder known as anorexia nervosa. Anorexics are controlled by a compulsive desire or need to lose weight. Most begin with modest dieting goals, but once

---

[18] Facts cited by Wayne Wooley in a speech delivered at the 1979 convention of the National Association to Aid Fat Americans *(see p. 75).*
[19] Quoted by Bennett and Gurin, *op. cit.,* p. 87.
[20] Quoted by Susan Edwards, *op. cit.,* p. 93.

started, they lose control and either refuse to or find they cannot stop. Many victims starve themselves to the point of serious illness or death.

There are differing theories about the causes of anorexia nervosa, but many experts attribute the problem to society's emphasis on beauty and thinness. Psychiatrist Hilda Bruch, considered a pioneer in the field of eating disorders, wrote:

> It is impossible to assess the cost in serenity, relaxation, and efficiency of this abnormal, overslim, fashionable appearance. It produces serious psychological tensions to feel compelled to be thinner than one's natural make-up and style of living demand. There is a great deal of talk about the weakness and self-indulgence of overweight people who eat "too much." Very little is said about the selfishness and self-indulgence involved in a life which makes one's appearance the center of all values, and subordinates all other considerations to it.[21]

Ideal Women's Figures Through History

The taut, thin body so prized and coveted by fashion designers, the media and most contemporary women has not always been as desirable as it is today. "Women's bodies have been a screen onto which different values have been projected by men: receptive sexiness and the promise of fecundity, in the main," Bennett and Gurin wrote. "For hundreds of years, these attributes were manifested in the fleshiness of the woman's figure." [22] In some cultures fleshiness is still considered desirable: in India, for example, a thin woman is often considered scrawny and her worth as a bearer of children — insurance for a comfortable old age — questionable.

Since about 1400, three types of women have been idealized in the West, according to social historians. The first was the reproductive woman, characterized by a prominent belly. Throughout the Middle Ages the ability to bear children was especially important to high-born women, and the capacity to produce an heir the criterion for marital success. Nudes in 15th and 16th century paintings often look pregnant, and women's clothing styles emphasized the stomach. Art historian Anne Hollander wrote in *Seeing Through Clothes* (1978) that "in the erotic imagination of Europe, it was apparently impossible until the late 17th century for a woman to have too big a belly."

In the 17th century the status of women began to shift. Upper-class families started limiting the number of children they produced and a chilly atmosphere of emotional isolation seemed to pervade family life. But by 1700 children and tender-

---

[21] Hilda Bruch, *Eating Disorders* (1973), p. 198.
[22] Bennett and Gurin, *op. cit.*, pp. 170-171.

ness toward them were rediscovered. "As a result of this warming emotional climate," Bennett and Gurin wrote, "a generation of articulate men was born, some of them artists, who had fond, not merely formal, memories of their mothers — and these memories could be worked into their erotic imaginations." The result was a revision of the ideal woman's body. The belly, symbol of female fertility, became de-emphasized and the body with ample breasts, hips and buttocks became the erotic ideal.

Also in the 18th century, women began to diet. Before that time the constant threat of famine made going voluntarily hungry absurd, but by the 1800s the English upper class, at least, had a secure food supply. Around this time pallor also became the rage, easily obtained through nutritional deprivation, enemas and purges. Wire bodices pinched in waists and pushed up breasts, and bustles made women's buttocks look huge. Some women even had their lower ribs removed to produce more of an hourglass shape.

By the latter part of the 19th century, women had taken up bicycling, roller skating, tennis and other sports. Vigorous activity and exercise were promoted for women, and clothing styles adapted to allow them more freedom of movement. The arrival of motion pictures in the 20th century conveyed women's new image for all to see. Movies became the main source of mass entertainment and have consistently, throughout this century, set trends in feminine beauty and desirability.

Mania for Thinness in the 20th Century

By the 1920s the birth control movement and women's suffrage — the two events that contributed most to women's liberation at the beginning of the century — were facts of life. In 1921 women's fashion introduced the slender silhouette, and the flapper was born. The stylish woman of the 1920s had bobbed hair, slender hips and legs and no breasts to speak of — either by natural endowment or because she bound them flat. The new woman was active — physically, socially and sexually.

In the 1940s and 1950s a more buxom ideal took hold — a reversion to the hourglass shape of earlier times — reflected in such movie stars as Jane Russell and Marilyn Monroe. Monroe was probably the last popular sex symbol to have a fleshy, sumptuous body. The lean body asserted itself with a vengeance in the 1960s. Ironically, while this decade witnessed the growth and development of feminism, it also produced a new fashion image of boyishness, adolescence and asexuality.

While some interpret slimness as an expression of power, albeit gained at great cost, Kay Chernin, a consultant to women with eating disorders in Berkeley, Calif., sees our culture's

71

obsession with slenderness as a fear of women's power, perhaps related to the almost mythic power of mothers experienced in infancy. "We have strong, ambivalent feelings about the relationship between a woman's power and her size, and they are reflected in our dislike for large fleshy women," Chernin wrote. "Thus the male-dominated culture calls for slender women, unconsciously seeking to limit the symbolic physical expression of their power. And women themselves accept this tyranny of slenderness because of their own ambivalence about their bodies."[23] Chernin believes that women obsessed with their body size must resolve the basic cultural conflicts they have internalized. "Fat or thin, voluptuous or lean, full or angular, a woman's authentic beauty first comes into existence when her body expresses her self-acceptance," she wrote in *The Obsession: Reflections on the Tyranny of Slenderness* (1981).

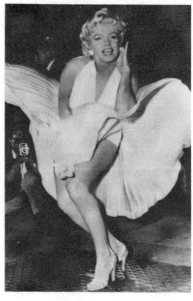

Marilyn Monroe

Weight Control Methods

WHILE some women — and men — have come to terms with their bodies, no matter what their weight, many are still frantically pursuing the cultural esthetic. This is probably fortunate only for the authors of diet books and entrepreneurs who develop new weight-loss schemes. But medical experts say many of the popular diets are dangerous. For example, the Beverly Hills Diet touted by Judy Mazel in her book of that name consists mainly of fruit and avoidance of protein for several weeks. According to neurologist Richard Restak, the book is filled with medical inaccuracies and its advice could lead to severe diarrhea, shock, and even irregular heartbeat.[24]

[23] Kay Chernin, "How Women's Diets Reflect Fear of Power," *The New York Times Magazine*, Oct. 11, 1981, p. 44.
[24] Richard Restak, "Medicine Avenue," *Science Digest*, May 1982, p. 38.

The newest rage is the Cambridge Diet, essentially a modified fast that consists of only 330 calories a day. Besides being dangerous if the dieter is not monitored carefully through regular electrocardiograms or blood tests, such modified fasts may be ineffective. "The body doesn't know it's fasting," said Aaron Altschul, head of the Georgetown University Diet Management Clinic. "It thinks it's starving, so it mobilizes its defenses to protect its fat stores, making it harder and harder for the weight to come off." [25]

Cambridge Diet literature now contains warnings against its use without strict medical supervision by those with hypertension, diabetes, heart or kidney problems, gout, hypoglycemia or by the elderly, growing children, pregnant women and nursing mothers. The literature also says that the diet should not be used without other sources of nutrition for more than a month or with medication like diuretics. But some people on the diet could have ailments of which they are not aware. The Food and Drug Administration (FDA) is investigating at least three cases of women who were hospitalized for heart irregularities as well as one death attributed to the diet.

More legitimate treatment for the overweight involves behavior modification. This approach is based on the idea that people need to change their lifestyles and eating habits to lose weight and keep it off. Patients who undergo behavior modification are first told to monitor and record their regular eating habits. Then, along with a therapist, they examine the account with a view toward locating the special circumstances, such as watching television, that encourage them to overeat.

Reliance on Pills and Other Substances

Eating less, exercising more, and changing eating habits are legitimate ways to try to lose weight, but the desperate sometimes depend on diet pills, notably amphetamines, to help kill uncooperative appetites. But amphetamines are powerful, habit-forming drugs with serious side effects. Not only are they widely abused, but their effectiveness as an appetite suppressant, particularly with prolonged use, has been questioned. To try to curb amphetamine abuse, the Justice Department about 10 years ago started limiting the drug's production. In July 1979 the Food and Drug Administration announced its intention to ban the use of amphetamines as a diet aid. But the proposed ban is still being contested by the drug's manufacturers.

Other drugs have come under government fire as well. On July 1, 1982, the FDA ordered a halt to the manufacture and sale of "starch blockers," which producers claimed allowed starch to pass through the body without being broken down and

---

[25] Quoted in *The Washington Post*, Oct. 15, 1982.

absorbed as calories. The FDA said it had received reports of adverse reactions to the pills, including vomiting, diarrhea, nausea and stomach pains. A group of starch blocker manufacturers filed suit against the agency, but on Oct. 5, the U.S. District Court in Chicago upheld the ban. The manufacturers have said they will appeal the ruling.

Dieters can still choose from a variety of over-the-counter diet pills, sold under such names as Dexatrim and Dietac. These pills have been selling briskly since 1979 when an FDA panel declared that their primary ingredient, phenylpropanolamine, may help some people lose weight.[26] Also effective as an appetite suppressant, the panel said, was benzocaine, a local anesthetic that numbs the tastebuds and which is sold to dieters in candy and chewing gum form.

Another drug now being studied by Eli Lilly Co. and at least two other drug companies would mimic the metabolic effects of exercise by burning up fat. Diet experts believe this weight loss method might produce serious side effects and, though intended only for the dangerously obese, would also be used by marginally overweight people looking for an easy way to slim down.

Other researchers have developed a synthetic fat that contains no calories and is reportedly indistinguishable from the real thing. Sucrose polyester — not related to the polyester in clothing — consists of a sucrose molecule attached to eight fatty acids. The fat passes through the body undigested and therefore is not absorbed as calories. According to Dr. Charles J. Glueck at the University of Cincinnati, initial findings indicate that sucrose polyester can help very obese people lose weight. Procter & Gamble holds the patent for it, but it could be years before the FDA approves it.

Those looking for ways to drop a few pounds by at least cutting out sugar from their diets may have an answer as close as their supermarket shelves. Aspartame is a new artificial sweetener that is virtually non-caloric, has no aftertaste and does not cause cancer in laboratory animals. It may be dangerous only to those with a rare genetic disease called phenylketonuria, and a warning label to this effect will appear on all products containing the sweetener.[27]

Improved Image of Overweight People

Increasingly, fat people and some thin people as well are rebelling against what many see as an exaggerated view of obesity's ill effects on health and against society's view that thin is good and beautiful and fat is bad and ugly. Clothing manufac-

[26] Recent evidence suggests that phenylpropanolamine may have some serious side-effects. See Bennet and Gurin, *op. cit.*, pp. 224-225.

[27] See Gene Bylinsky, "The Battle for America's Sweet Tooth," *Fortune*, July 26, 1982.

Exercise: Key to Weight Control

Many experts believe exercise is the key to losing weight and keeping it off and much of the public apparently agrees. Over half of all Americans now participate in some form of daily physical exercise, according to a recent *Washington Post*-ABC News public opinion poll. "In the past 20 years the number of American adults who exercise regularly has continued to increase," C. Carson Conrad, executive director of the President's Council on Physical Fitness and Sports, told the *Post*. "And it hasn't peaked."

One of the most important trends in the physical fitness craze is the marked increase in women sports participants. The Post-ABC poll found that more men exercise regularly than women, but women may be catching up. About 60 percent of the men surveyed said they exercised daily, compared to 46 percent of the women.

The poll also found that an increasing number of senior citizens are becoming active in sports and exercise programs. About 40 percent of those over age 60 said they exercised daily, compared to two-thirds of those between 18 and 30.

Those who need to exercise most seem to have the most trouble sticking to an exercise regime. More than 30 perent of obese persons drop out of physical exercise programs, according to Professor Kelly D. Brownell of the University of Pennsylvania.

Overweight people are often told to exercise because it burns off calories, but the amount of calories burned is relatively small compared to the amount of energy expended. On the other hand, exercise does seem to reduce appetite and to offset the decrease in metabolism that occurs when people diet. Exercise also counteracts some of the physical and psychological effects of extreme overweight — such as high blood pressure, low self-esteem and depression — even if weight loss does not occur.

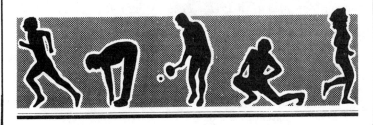

turers are making more clothes in large sizes and magazines such as *BBW* — for big beautiful women — offer beauty and fashion advice for "full-figured" women. Books such as *Big and Beautiful* (1982) by Ruthanne Olds advise readers to stop dieting and start living.

The National Association to Aid Fat Americans was founded in 1969 by engineer William Fabrey to promote self-esteem and equal rights for fat Americans.[28] The group holds meetings, lectures and social events, publishes a newsletter and sponsors some obesity research. "We do nothing to promote or discourage weight loss," Fabrey said last year, but sometimes people who join NAAFA lose weight unintentionally when they start respecting themselves and thinking about other things besides their weight.[29]

"Obesity is a predicament of people in affluent societies," Dr. Theodore Van Itallie told *Psychology Today.* "So much of what we do and think is determined by factors we haven't reflected on or mastered — such as the nature of our diet, the constant display of advertised temptations, the dependence on cars, and the absence of sidewalks. Maybe the next generation will pay more attention to them and learn to control them." In the meantime, experts advise that society's understanding could go a long way in easing unnecessary stress and low self-esteem in overweight people.

[28] The group's address is P.O. Box 43, Bellerose, N.Y. 11426.
[29] Quoted in *NAAFA 'Extra,* no. 4, 1982.

Selected Bibliography

Books

Bennett, William and Joel Gurin, *The Dieter's Dilemma,* Basic Books, 1982.

Bruch, Hilda, *Eating Disorders,* Basic Books, 1973.

Chernin, Kay, *The Obsession: Reflections on the Tyranny of Slenderness,* Harper Colophon Books, 1981.

Edwards, Susan, *Too Much is Not Enough,* McGraw-Hill, 1981.

Millman, Marcia, *Such a Pretty Face: Being Fat in America,* W. W. Norton & Co., 1980.

Stunkard, Albert, ed., *Obesity,* W. B. Saunders, 1980.

Articles

Anderegg, Karen, "Are We Fatness Crazy?" *Vogue,* March 1982.

Brownell, Kelly D., "Obesity: Understanding and Treating a Serious, Prevalent, and Refractory Disorder," *Journal of Consulting and Clinical Psychology,* no. 6, vol. 50, March 1982.

"Conspiracy Against Fatness," *Psychology Today,* October 1978.

Journal of the American Medical Association, selected issues.

Van Itallie, Theodore, "Obesity: The American Disease," *Food Technology,* December 1979.

Reports and Studies

Abraham, Sidney and Clifford L. Johnson, "Overweight Adults in the United States," National Center for Health Statistics, 1979.

Editorial Research Reports: "Obesity and Health," 1977 Vol. I, p. 453; "Physical Fitness Boom," 1978 Vol. I, pp. 261-180.

MENTAL HEALTH CARE REAPPRAISAL

by

William Sweet

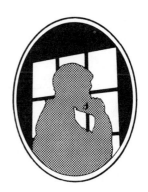

**Aug. 20
1 9 8 2**

Editor's Note: Bills to restrict the application of the insanity defense in federal courts *(see p. 98)* were introduced in Congress last year, but none won final approval. A provision limiting the insanity defense was included in a bill approved by the Senate Judiciary Committee on July 21, 1983, to simplify and modernize federal criminal laws. The measure would limit the insanity defense to those defendants who could prove, by clear and convincing evidence, that they were unable to appreciate the wrongfulness of their acts. The proposal would shift the burden of proof from the prosecutor, who currently must show beyond a reasonableness doubt that the defendant does not meet the insanity test. The House Judiciary Subcommittee on Criminal Justice, on June 16, approved an insanity bill that includes a definition of insanity that is almost identical to the Senate's, but it would require the defendant to prove his insanity claim only by a preponderance of evidence — a lesser test than the "clear and convincing" evidence standard in the Senate bill.

MENTAL HEALTH CARE
REAPPRAISAL

THE REMOVAL of mentally ill people from large institutions and their placement into community situations is not a new story, but it remains, even after a quarter-century of steady deinstitutionalization, a deeply troubling story. Just about everybody involved in the process describes the results as unsatisfactory, or worse.

What was justified as an effort to provide disturbed people with more humane treatment in less restrictive settings has left thousands of patients adrift, barely able or unable to cope, and for thousands more it has meant re-institutionalization in inappropriate facilities. The comprehensive system of community care facilities that was supposed to take the place of central institutions is only half-built, and now, at a time when federal programs are being cut, professionals in the mental health field are beginning to wonder whether deinstitutionalization was a mistake.

Since the late 1960s, yearly spending on community care facilities has increased enormously. By 1978, the latest year for which figures have been officially compiled, spending was above $1 billion and more than two million patients were receiving help in such facilities annually. The number of patients in mental hospitals dropped to less than 150,000 from a peak of about 650,000 in the mid-1950s.

Hundreds of thousands of people have not really been deinstitutionalized, however. Instead, they have been transferred to nursing homes, where they may be getting less professional care than they had in their original institutional settings. As for the people who really have been deinstitutionalized, thousands are receiving inadequate care in the community or no care at all. Of the 1,500-2,500 community mental health facilities anticipated in federal legislation passed in 1963 *(see p. 93)*, fewer than 800 have been built, and they serve only about half of the U.S. nation.

In cities all over the country — New York, Washington, Detroit, Portland, Ore., San Francisco, Dallas — disturbed, homeless people have become a familiar sight on the streets. To the untrained eye, most of these people look like mere degenerates. But to anybody who has seen the inside of an institution, many of the derelicts are readily recognizable as veterans of mental wards. On the streets, they often are attired in the bizarre and outlandish ways that inmates adopt to distinguish themselves from their fellows in the drab, monotonous atmosphere of a crowded institution. Like people confined to wards, they have their meager possessions in string bags, clinging to whatever they can find to enhance their sense of identity and character.

In congressional testimony last May, Eleanor Owen, vice president of the National Alliance for the Mentally Ill, said that "we now have 750,000 mentally ill in nursing homes, 110,000 in short-term psychiatric hospitals, hundreds of thousands living in 'group homes' . . . and thousands sleeping in alleys and missions. Still others are shuffled through the costly criminal justice system. . . . In the last decade, there has been a 300 percent increase in the arrest rate of the mentally ill." [1] Owen drew attention especially to the situation of the severely or chronically mentally ill. "We have spent billions of dollars, developed a vast community mental health system and yet, data show, we have neither 'deinstitutionalized,' nor rehabilitated, nor improved the quality of life for the chronically mentally ill," she said.

C. Bernard Smith, executive director of the alliance, has called deinstitutionalization a "disaster" — a "quick, simple solution" taken for dubious political and economic reasons." [2] There are "very few communities," Smith said, that can boast "adequate comprehensive services," such as 24-hour crisis assistance, programs to monitor drug prescription and use, clinical support, housing, vocational and social rehabilitation, etc.

The National Alliance for the Mentally Ill is just one of the groups that has sought to draw attention to the plight of mentally ill people in nursing homes and in the streets. The American Federation of State, County and Municipal Employees (AFSCME), which represents about a quarter of a million workers in mental institutions and institutions for the retarded, has run ads in national publications denouncing the way mentally ill people are being treated in the community. An ad it placed in a socialist newsweekly in 1980 focused on a mentally ill man who allegedly died because of incorrect diagnosis and neglect in a nursing home: "Everybody wanted the best for Dan Radovsky," the headline of the ad read. "That's what killed him." [3]

Last May, Robert M. Hayes of the Coalition for the Homeless

---

[1] Testimony on fiscal year 1983 mental health research, training and services, Senate Appropriations Committee, Subcommittee on Labor, Health and Human Services, May 5, 1982.
[2] Interview, June 23, 1982.
[3] See *In These Times* (Chicago), Nov. 5-11, 1980, pp. 16-17.

Growth of Community Care System

Year	Number of Community Care Centers	Number of Patients Under Care	Number of Outpatient Visits
1968	165	271,590	n.a.
1969	205	373,097	n.a.
1970	255	517,661	2,839,664
1971	295	693,260	3,375,705
1972	325	846,336	3,902,716
1973	400	1,094,430	5,202,016
1974	434	1,322,832	6,055,759
1975	528	1,618,746	7,596,434
1976	548	1,877,676	8,669,115
1977	563	1,881,798	8,934,220
1978	600	2,136,711	9,724,305

Source: National Institute of Mental Health

filed suit against New York state on behalf of the mentally ill in New York City's streets. Of the 40,000 homeless people estimated to be living in the city, as many as half may be mentally ill. Hayes' suit, which asked the court to order the state to provide residences for the homeless ill, was hailed as a constructive step by Mayor Edward I. Koch and City Council President Carol Bellamy. On Aug. 11, the New York Mental Health Information Service brought suit against the state on behalf of 140 mental patients in the Manhattan State Psychiatric Center. The Information Service, a legal aid group associated with the State Supreme Court's Appellate Division, claims that the patients are being confined because there is no place in the community for them to go and it asks the state to provide community shelters.

Last Dec. 28 an activist group in Washington called the Community for Creative Non-Violence planted 539 crosses in Lafayette Park, across Pennsylvania Avenue from the White House. Each cross represented a homeless person who had died of neglect during the previous five years in 11 areas where relevant statistics are compiled. In the United States as a whole, there are thought to be between a quarter of a million and one million homeless people, many of them emotionally disturbed.

Funding Cuts, Block Grants, SSI Review

Despite efforts on behalf of the mentally ill, the trend since 1980 has been to reduce federal funding and relax federal standards for community programs. The new national policies represent a marked reversal of measures adopted during the Carter presidency when first lady Rosalynn Carter took a personal interest in mental health care issues and served as chairperson of a special presidential commission.[4]

In February 1978, a task force connected with President Carter's Commission on Mental Health issued a report in which it referred to the "chronically mentally disabled" as "politically and economically powerless" people who "rarely speak for themselves." [5] The panel went on to say that "deinstitutionalization has too often occurred without adequate planning. It has too frequently been propelled by a desire to shift fiscal responsibility from the states to the federal government and has proceeded on unverified assumptions that appropriate community care for these people exists."

The work of the presidential commission contributed to the enactment by Congress in 1980 of the Mental Health Systems Act. The bill authorized increased federal funding for mental health services over a five-year period. Starting in 1982, outlays were to be targeted at specially disadvantaged groups such as the elderly, severely disturbed children and the chronically mentally ill. While the bill increased the state role in distribution of federal funds, it also included safeguards to protect the interests of community centers.

Following President Reagan's election, Congress in effect repealed most of the 1980 law and the Community Mental Health Facilities Act of 1963 by block-granting federal funds for the mentally ill. While 1981 legislation provided some guarantees for continued funding of community centers that were already being phased in, it gave states much greater discretion in disposing of federal funds. In addition, overall federal funding for mental health programs was cut roughly 25 percent in 1982, and the Reagan budget plans anticipate continued funding at the lower level in the years ahead. On Aug. 10, House and Senate conferees agreed on $12.5 billion in cuts over three years in Medicare, Medicaid and welfare programs, including reductions in health funding for the elderly and disabled.

Advocates for the mentally ill complain that their constituents already are being adversely affected by the Reagan administration's accelerated review of social security rolls, which was called for in 1980 legislation. Some 4.5 million Americans receive benefits under the Social Security Disability Insurance and Supplemental Security Income programs. Evidently, the administration plans to review over 500,000 recipients in fiscal 1982 and save $200 million by reducing the rolls — many of them people who have been classified as mentally disabled.

---

[4] See "Mental Health Care," *E.R.R.*, 1979 Vol. II, pp. 683-685.

[5] "Report of the Task Panel on Deinstitutionalization, Rehabilitation and Long-Term Care," Feb. 15, 1978.

Mental Health Care Reappraisal

A coalition of groups that includes the Association for Retarded Citizens, the Mental Health Law Project and National Alliance for the Mentally Ill has denounced the roll review as a "misguided" way to save money. The coalition argues that many people removed from the rolls will be unable to support themselves without federal assistance and will end up in hospitals, resulting ultimately in greater costs to federal, state and local governments.[6] In New York state alone the denial rate is reported to be 44 percent, and if this rate is sustained, over 70,000 people could lose their social security benefits over the next two years.[7]

Another Reagan administration measure opposed by mental health groups is a proposed regulation that would reduce enforcement of standards for nursing homes. The Department of Health and Human Services proposal would eliminate the requirement for annual inspection and allow many homes to be inspected only every other year, and it would allow states to turn over certification to the Joint Commission on Accreditation of Hospitals, an industry group funded by the facilities it inspects.[8]

On the defensive, mental health groups have struggled to protect the fledgling Community Support Program. The experimental CSP program, established in the 1980 mental health act, has provided about $7 million annually to 19 state agencies to assess delivery systems, identify service gaps, recommend how resources should be reallocated, and evaluate new approaches. It is somewhat similar to the measures in the 1975 Developmental Disabilities Act that provided for the establishment in every state of Developmental Disability Councils to assess delivery systems for mentally handicapped people.[9]

Uneven Services and Lack of Coordination

The adequacy of mental health services is extremely difficult to assess on a national scale because systems vary drastically among regions and states and even within individual states. Specialists generally agree that problems are most acute in the industrial Northeastern states because they had the largest institutional populations, often were the first to deinstitutionalize and now have the largest numbers of displaced people on the streets. Dr. Aaron Lieberman, executive director of the National Council of Community Mental Health

---

[6] See Mental Health Law Project, "Arbitrary Reduction of Disability Rolls," 1982, p. 3.
[7] See Stephen S. Hall, "When Bureaucracy Meets Madness," *The Village Voice*, Aug. 10, 1982, p. 21.
[8] See *The Nation*, July 24-31, 1982, p. 69, and Mental Health Law Project, "Update," June 22, 1982. Also see "Housing Options for the Elderly," *E.R.R.*, 1982 Vol. II, pp. 574-576.
[9] Not all the recent news has been bad news for the mentally ill. Section 2176 of last year's Budget Reconciliation Act included an important new waiver to the Medicaid program for "home and community based services" which will make it easier for disabled people outside institutions to get federal benefits for non-medical needs such as housing.

Centers, said in an interview that New York state and New York City especially have "dreadful problems." [10] In Massachusetts and Michigan, he said, recessionary pressures are sorely straining health care budgets; in the West, the same is true in Washington state and — because of Proposition 13, the balanced-budget initiative — in California.[11] As examples of states that have "extremely well-developed" community care services, Lieberman mentioned Arkansas, North Carolina, Missouri, Texas and Oregon.

Even in some of these states, services reportedly leave a lot to be desired. In Texas, according to a story in the *Dallas Times Herald* this year:

- "The community clinics and other services envisioned under the deinstitutionalization movement have turned out to be empty promises. . . ."

- "About 75 percent of Texas' health care budget goes for the 20 percent of the mentally ill and mentally retarded who are in institutions, while only 20 percent goes for the 80 percent who are served by community programs. . . ."

- In 1981, "2,000 Dallas County residents were released from state hospitals to return to an area where there are only 103 slots in halfway houses, supervised apartments or lodges. . . ."

- ". . . [M]any patients have nowhere to go. By several estimates, they make up one-third of the derelicts who live on the streets and in the alleys of Dallas. . . ."

- ". . . [F]ormer mental patients are landing in jails and prisons at an alarming rate. . . ."

- "Increasingly, unlicensed private boarding homes have become virtual warehouses for the mentally ill, many of them elderly persons abandoned by their families." [12]

Willamette Week reported last October that the situation is similar in Multnomah County, Ore., home of Portland. There are estimated to be 6,000 chronically mentally ill people in the county — most of them single, under 35 and unemployed. The county, according to *Willamette Week,* has "only one group home for the chronically ill with a capacity of 15 — men only. It has no other halfway houses or apartments." [13]

Rarely, even in the best service systems, has there been any provision for the systematic transfer of funds and personnel from central institutions to community care facilities, as pa-

---

[10] Interview, June 28, 1982.

[11] Even though California is given credit for having one of the nation's better mental health care systems, attorneys for the Mental Health Association in California filed suit in February 1979 against Gov. Edmund G. (Jerry) Brown Jr. for "failure to set up adequate community services" for thousands of mental patients "unnecessarily" confined to institutions.

[12] Linda Austin, "The Mental Health Care Crisis: How the System Failed," *Dallas Times Herald,* May 30, 1982.

[13] Phil Keisling, "The Empty Asylum," *Willamette Week,* Oct. 20-26, 1981. Keisling is now an editor of the *Washington Monthly* in Washington, D.C.

tients have been deinstitutionalized. The two systems often are run by separate agencies, each with its own vested interests. Directors of central institutions, the communities that depend on them for employment and revenue, and labor unions all resist closures or reductions in staffing and budgets.

Partly for this reason, the number of central institutions and the number of people working in them have remained essentially unchanged for the last 30 years. Since the number of patients in the institutions has dropped sharply, per capita hospitalization costs have soared: Daily hospitalization costs in psychiatric facilities went from $5 in 1960 to $75 in 1979, far faster than the general rate of inflation.[14] Considering how overcrowded institutions were to begin with and how underpaid their staffs have been, the higher expenditures may be justified. But they are a drain, just the same, on funds available for community care systems.

Plight of Revolving-Door Mental Patients

Funding for community care programs comes from a very wide range of sources *(see box, p. 87)*, and frequently regulations and instruction do too. Rarely is there any one person or agency responsible for coordinating all the services a discharged mental patient needs: psychiatric counseling; prescription and monitoring of drugs; help with employment problems; residential supervision; assistance in obtaining benefits to which individuals may be entitled; and social rehabilitation aid. The result, too often, is that patients either get lost altogether or go through a bewildering series of therapies in and out of institutions.

Harry Schnibbe, director of the National Association of State Mental Health Program Directors, has taken the position that mental health programs cannot be expected to assume responsibility for all the problems discharged patients have. He said that providing jobs for such people is a "welfare issue," not a "health care issue."[15] When people are discharged from institutions, Schnibbe said, they are "cured" or "able to cope."

Most independent specialists emphatically disagree with the view that a mental health agency's responsibilities end when a patient is discharged. The precipitous decrease during the past two and a half decades in the number of patients permanently confined to institutions has been accompanied by huge increases in the number of revolving-door patients who are in and out of hospitals.[16] The typical patient discharged from a hos-

---

[14] Bureau of the Census, *Statistical Abstract* (1981), p. 111. In that time the Consumer Price Index increased 163 percent — more than doubling but short of tripling 1960 prices.
[15] Interview, June 18, 1982.
[16] See Ellen L. Bassuk, and Samuel Gerson, "Deinstitutionalization and Mental Health Services," *Scientific American*, February 1978, pp. 43-53.

pital has turned out to need some form of continuing care, and many need to be re-hospitalized periodically for intensive treatment.

In a widely noted series that appeared in *The New Yorker* magazine in 1981 and as a book this year, Susan Sheehan described the experiences of one revolving-door patient — given the fictional name "Sylvia Frumkin" — in a remarkably large number of New York institutions and community programs.[17] It is a story of contradictory diagnoses, often by doctors who did not speak English very well and who did not trouble themselves to study her case records; erratic and confusing therapeutic advice by counselors, family and friends; misguided and often counterproductive drug prescriptions; and a general behavioral deterioration that seemed to get worse the more care Frumkin got. "Is there no place on earth for me?" Frumkin took to asking — a lament that provided the title for Sheehan's book.

Talk of Returning to Central Institutions

Robert Herman, director of the National Mental Health Association, remains convinced that "deinstitutionalization is good if it's not capricious." [18] Like many other people involved in mental health care, Herman believes that disturbed people will eventually get better treatment if they are kept visible in the community than they received when they were isolated from public view in state hospitals. "The whole problem" with mental health care, Herman said, is that "it's always somebody else's problem."

Writers on mental health topics have found many instances around the country of well-run community programs. The ones most frequently mentioned include Montana's Community Support Project; Training in Community Living in Madison, Wis.; Fairweather Lodges in Texas; Fountain House in New York City; and Green Door in Washington, D.C.[19] Moreover, it seems to be true, Jean Elshtain wrote in *The Nation* last year, that discharged patients "almost to a person ... say that despite all the 'hassles' and inadequate facilities on the 'outside,' they prefer this 'least restrictive' environment to that most restrictive of all, the total institution." [20]

Regrettably, the fact that patients express greater happiness in the community does not necessarily mean that they are getting more effective treatment than they would in hospitals. Two studies of community programs in northwestern Illinois

---

[17] Susan Sheehan, *Is There No Place on Earth for Me?* (1982).
[18] Interview, July 22, 1982.
[19] See Samantha Grove Johnson, "Health Care's Dumping Ground," *The Boston Globe Magazine*, May 30, 1982, p. 16.
[20] Jean Bethke Elshtain, "A Key to Unlock the Asylum?" *The Nation*, May 16, 1981, p. 603.

Funding for Federally Aided Community Mental Health Centers, 1978

Source of Funds	Total (add 000)	Percent	Average Per center (add 000)
Total receipts from all sources	$1,274,386	100.0%	$2,124
Government funds	816,226	64.2	1,360
Federal funds	270,371	21.2	451
Staffing grants	193,272	15.2	322
Construction grants	10,007	0.8	17
Children's grants	18,091	1.4	30
Research and training	4,934	0.4	8
Other federal funds	44,068	3.5	73
State funds	431,662	33.9	719
Local government funds	112,148	8.8	187
Other government funds	2,043	0.2	3
Receipts from direct services	405,320	31.8	676
Patient fees	47,309	3.7	79
Insurance (private or voluntary)	93,151	7.3	155
Medicare	37,288	2.9	62
Medicaid	139,383	10.9	232
From schools	12,290	1.0	20
Title XX	47,298	3.7	79
Other receipts from services	28,601	2.2	48
Receipts from indirect services	7,288	0.6	12
Schools	2,425	0.2	4
Other	4,862	0.4	8
Philanthropy	6,848	0.5	11
Other fund raising	10,871	0.8	18
Other receipts	27,836	2.2	46
Number of Centers	600		

Sums may vary from stated totals because of rounding.

Source: National Institute of Mental Health

found the results ambiguous. "In the first study there was no indication," the authors said, "that community care was superior to that of a traditional state hospital. Seventy-four percent of the patients in the sample, however, had a history of repeated hospitalizations. The second study evaluated only first-admission patients and found that community-oriented programs were more effective." [21]

The authors found in the first study that total health care

---

[21] See W. G. Smith and D. W. Hart, "Community Mental Health: A Noble Failure?" *Hospital and Community Psychiatry*, September 1975, p. 581.

costs were higher in the community than in the institution. Also, they discovered that in northwestern Illinois — like many other parts of the country — deinstitutionalization was something of a myth. Of 1,200 people in state hospitals in 1966, "more than 70 percent of the original group are still in some form of institutional care — hospitals, nursing homes or extended care facilities." [22]

In light of their findings, the authors wondered "how close is the day when someone re-invents the state hospital — a well-run place in the clear country air where the disabled can be cared for humanely and money can be saved by buying necessities in bulk lots." In a similar vein, Dr. Leona Bachrach, a sociologist with the National Institute for Mental Health, has argued in a series of papers that the range of functions performed by hospitals is more complex and harder to duplicate in the community than once was thought. "In the zeal of reform," Bachrach wrote, "deinstitutionalization efforts have, in practice, too often confused locus of care with quality of care." [23]

Locating the Outcast Ill

IN MEDIEVAL EUROPE, it was common practice to confine mad people in the city gates, where they could be seen behind iron grills by anybody entering or leaving the walled communities. The gates, at the boundary of civilization and wilderness, safety and insecurity, were a fitting place for people who were regarded at that time as hybrid creatures — part human and part beast, or part devil and part divine.

The confinement of the insane at "the point of passage," between the known world and mysterious beyond, reached a culmination in the late Middle Ages when "ships of fools" carried loads of lunatics from city to city on the rivers and seas of continental Europe.[24] Very likely, the ships were used to deport unwanted vagrants — medieval bag people, who apparently drifted to the more livable cities, just as they do today. But the ships also figured large in the popular imagination, as one element in what became a virtual obsession with madness at the close of the Middle Ages.

During the 15th century, according to the French social theorist Michel Foucault, a "dance of fools" displaced the tra-

[22] *Ibid.*, p. 583.
[23] Leona L. Bachrach, "A Conceptual Approach to Deinstitutionalization," *Hospital and Community Psychiatry*, September 1978, p. 577.
[24] See Michel Foucault, *Madness and Civilization* (1965), p. 11.

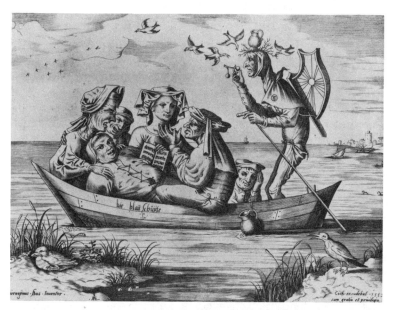

"Ship of Fools" by Hieronymus Bosch, 1559

ditional dance of death in popular festivals. In the dance of fools, Foucault speculated, the people of that time acted out "the dizzying unreason of the world." It was as though, at the dawn of the age of reason, a consciousness of absurdity in life was replacing a preoccupation with the end of life.[25]

Perhaps too, at a time when religious authority was weakening, and when people were beginning to imagine a social order based on man's sovereign aspirations, madness embodied the twin threats of unreason and perversity — "temptation," in Foucault's words, or the "freedom, however frightening, of dreams." If so, the collective response seems to have been what psychologists now call "denial." During the following centuries, madness disappeared from popular rituals as a major theme, and the insane increasingly were isolated in large institutions.

In 1547, the Bethlehem Royal Hospital in London, popularly known as Bedlam, was converted at the orders of Henry VIII into an insane asylum. This was one of the first institutions in Europe to be established exclusively for the custody of the mentally ill, and for centuries to come this kind of facility was more the exception than the rule. More often, in England as well as on the European continent, deranged people were thrown together with other vagrants of every description in work houses. These were created by secularizing monarchs and city councils, in the spirit of the emergent work ethic, to get

[25] In Foucault's words, consciousness of "that necessity which inevitably reduces man to nothing" shifted "to the scornful contemplation of that nothing which is existence itself." *Ibid.*, pp. 15-16.

undesirables off the streets and force them to contribute to the general economy.

In England, a law in 1575 called for the establishment in every county of "houses of correction" for the "punishment of vagabonds" and the "relief of the poor." During the following century, virtually every sizable German city set up similar facilities, the so-called *"Zuchthäuser."* In Paris, there was founded in 1656 the Hôpital Général, and within four years, its La Salpêtriére complex housed 1,460 vagabond beggers and its Bicêtre compound 1,615. Almost one tenth of these people apparently were insane, and because of their inability to adjust to the rigors of collective life, they typically fell victim to the "stakes, irons, prisons and dungeons" with which the Hôpital's superintendent was equipped by royal decree.

In colonial America the situation was little different. Mentally ill people usually were committed to alms houses, where they received no special treatment and sometimes were subject to the worst kind of abuse. Occasionally communities locked up the violently insane in improvised facilities, such as shacks erected on the commons. Generally, colonial governments passed laws for the expulsion of vagrants from other colonies or for their punitive confinement in work houses. The only institution established exclusively for the mentally ill in pre-Revolutionary America was founded in Williamsburg, Va., in 1766.

Rise and Fall of the 'Well-Ordered Institution'

By the end of the 18th century, many mentally ill people lived like zoo animals in cages, without clothes or sanitary facilities, often chained to the walls, with nothing but straw for warmth, comfort and hygiene. In some communities in France and England, it was a popular pastime for families to visit the local asylum on weekends, where parents and children would pay an admission fee for the pleasure of watching the mad act crazy. From the semi-divine, semi-human creature of the medieval imagination, the madman had been reduced to beast. And yet, in the act of isolating and debasing the madman, attention also was focused on him as a very special being with unique problems. It would be the task of a revolutionary era to attempt, however unsatisfactorily, his treatment and rehumanization.

In 1794, at the height of France's Revolution, the reforming physician Philippe Pinel (1745-1826) took the unprecedented step of unchaining the mad inmates of Bicêtre. As chief physician at Bicêtre and La Salpêtriére, Pinel made himself during the following decades the world's foremost proponent of more humane care for the insane, and he developed simple psychological methods of encouraging disturbed people to act more reasonably.

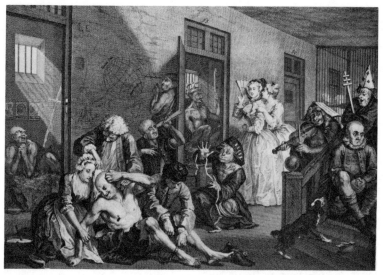

18th century madhouse portrayed by Hogarth in "The Rake's Progress"

In England, a Quaker family named Tuke played a similar role in designing retreats, in which they sought to remove deranged people from disruptive social influences and to reconstruct around them a wholesome environment similar to a community of Friends.[26] The corresponding part in America was played by Benjamin Rush (1745-1813), the Pennsylvania physician-patriot who wrote the first major work in this country on mental illness.[27]

The image of Pinel freeing insane people from their chains had "an immediate and obvious appeal" to the people of the new North American republic, according to Columbia University historian David J. Rothman, the leading authority on the development of the asylum in the United States.[28] During the period of Jacksonian reform, advocates of Pinel's "moral treatment" successfully campaigned to make it the standard method.

The 1820s and 1830s were a time of rapid social change in the United States, and among contemporary specialists on mental illness it was widely believed that insanity was a symptom of social stress. While specialists generally agreed that mental illness was a brain disease (even though the exact physical causes could not be explained), they tended to think that people would fall prey to insanity only when social causes were present. They thought, in particular, that the new republic's free society encouraged excessive ambitions and desires in many individ-

---

[26] William Tuke (1732-1822), the English pioneer in developing humane treatment for the insane, saw his work continued by his son Henry (1755-1814) and his grandson Samuel (1784-1857).

[27] *Inquiries and Observations Upon the Diseases of the Mind* (1812).

[28] David J. Rothman, *The Discovery of the Asylum* (1971), p. 110.

uals, and that these often were indulged too much by their families. The solution, in their view, was to subject the disturbed individual to the strict routine of the "well-ordered institution." Thus, the asylum came to be accepted as the preferred method of caring for the mentally ill.

In the typical institution of the 1830s and 1840s, discipline was stern but not cruel. The whip and chain were abolished, and the use of physical restraints was minimized. But contacts with family, friends and members of the wider community were discouraged, since they were seen as a source of the patient's problems. The superintendents of asylums, who liked to view themselves as benign despots, sought and gained absolute authority over the admission, treatment and discharging of their wards. In 1844, the superintendents formed a professional society, and in their publications they often made incredibly extravagant claims for their methods.[29] Some said they could cure all of their patients, using Pinel's methods.

The person who most embodied the utopian ideals behind the movement for asylums was Dorothea Dix (1802-1887). She went from state to state investigating the condition of the insane in poorhouses, jails and other institutions. "Her formula," Rothman wrote, "was simple and she repeated it everywhere: first assert the curability of insanity, link it directly to proper institutional care and then quote prevailing medical opinion on rates of recovery." [30] Dix is credited with having mobilized support for the creation of some 30 asylums. By the time of the Civil War, 28 of the nation's 33 states had established mental hospitals.

After the Civil War, a more cynical mood took hold, and by the 1870s, when Dix was completing her life's work, society was losing faith in the ideas and claims that had justified the creation of the asylum. Cure rates were unimpressive, and institutional care seemed too expensive in terms of the results achieved. State legislatures began to cut funding for asylums, without actually abolishing them. The institutions soon turned into purely custodial facilities, where people were warehoused under increasingly appalling conditions. The absolute authority of the superintendent remained intact, but with the idealism of the earlier years dead, the moral treatment was transformed into a harsh and mechanical discipline, dependent on the straitjackets and chains that once had been eliminated. The word "snakepits" came to characterize institutions for the insane, just as "bedlam" did in an earlier time.

---

[29] The Association of Medical Superintendents published the *American Journal of Insanity.* It ceased publication in July 1921 and was followed by the *American Journal of Psychiatry,* published by the American Psychiatric Association, successor to the Association of Medical Superintendents.

[30] David J. Rothman, *op. cit.*, p. 132.

"By the end of the century," two scholars have written, "the network of state mental hospitals, once a proud tribute to an era of reform, had largely turned into a bureaucratic morass within which patients were interned, often neglected and sometimes abused. That was the general situation [until] after World War II, when social, economic and medical developments prompted a reassessment of the delivery of psychiatric services." [31]

Impact of War, Drugs and Federal Money

World War II drew attention to the plight of the mentally ill and stimulated new thinking about alternatives to large-scale institutional care. Large numbers of draftees were rejected for psychiatric reasons, and many more cracked up under the strain of combat or training. New crisis-intervention and rehabilitation techniques were devised during the war, including the "quarter-way house," in which "shell-shock" victims would be treated within earshot of the front. After the war, still more servicemen needed psychiatric treatment, and as a result public attention was drawn to the primitive state of the nation's mental health care system. In 1946, Congress passed the National Mental Health Act, which established the National Institute of Mental Health to study the causes of mental illness and develop prevention strategies.

During the mid-1950s, the introduction of psychotropic drugs — chemicals that modify moods, thought processes and behavior — opened the way for a revolution in mental health care. Drugs like Thorazine proved to have a remarkably calming effect on many mental patients, and while such drugs have been very hard to prescribe in the right doses and combinations, their use made it possible to relax ward disciplinary systems and to discharge the most responsive patients into the community. In New York, for example, the amount of physical restraint and seclusion employed in the state institutions dropped 50 percent between the spring of 1955, when drugs were introduced, and the spring of 1956. The population confined in New York's state hospitals has declined steadily since 1955, when it peaked.

Another major development in 1955 was the creation by Congress of the Joint Commission on Mental Illness and Health. The commission's recommendations in 1960 provided the basis for a number of important initiatives by President Kennedy, which led in 1963 to enactment of the Mental Retardation Facilities and Community Mental Health Center Act. The legislation provided federal funding for community centers, which were to provide comprehensive services and individual case management for areas of 75,000 to 200,000 people.

---

[31] Ellen L. Bassuk and Samuel Gerson, *op. cit.*, p. 47.

The deinstitutionalization movement received yet another boost in 1965 with the enactment by Congress of Medicare and Medicaid. Patients in state hospitals under the age of 65 were excluded from Medicaid payments because funding for mental asylums had always been the responsibility of the states. The result of the Medicaid exclusion was that many states simply transferred patients to nursing homes, where they would be eligible for federal benefits. The Supplemental Security Income program, which was enacted in 1972, also excluded state hospital inmates and gave states an incentive to discharge patients into community settings.

Rights Revolution and Critique of Asylums

The enactment of federal entitlement programs coincided with the movement to guarantee full civil rights to black citizens, and it was not long before this movement broadened to encompass the concerns of other disadvantaged groups, including mentally ill people. A number of significant scholarly and literary works helped pave the way for this development. In one influential book, *Asylums* (1961), Erving Goffman provided a highly critical view of life in what he called "total institutions" — "places of residence" where "like-situated individuals" lead a segregated, "enclosed, formally administered round of life." The term total institution evoked images of concentration camps, and Goffman left the reader in no doubt about his partisan sympathy for the mental patient, whom he tended to portray as a victim of social type-casting.[32]

The same year *Asylums* appeared, Michel Foucault — the French social theorist, who holds degrees in philosophy, psychology and psychopathology — published his first major work, *Histoire de la Folie (Madness and Civilization* in its English language version). Like Goffman, Foucault wrote both as an accredited scholar and as a committed social critic. He opened his book with a telling quotation from Dostoyevsky: "It is not by confining one's own neighbor that one is convinced of one's own sanity." With that, Foucault announced his plans to "write the history of that other form of madness, by which men, in an act of sovereign reason, confine their neighbors, and communicate and recognize each other through the merciless language of non-madness; to define the moment of this conspiracy before it was permanently established in the realm of truth...."

Foucault probably has had little influence outside of academic circles. But ideas similar to his and Goffman's — the notion of institutionalization as a social conspiracy or a form of

---

[32] In one essay, Goffman said that "craziness or 'sick behavior' claimed for the mental patient is largely a product of the claimant's social distance from the situation that the patient is in, and is not primarily a product of mental illness." *Asylums* (1961), p. 130.

scapegoating, the image of the ward attendant as concentration camp guard — also manifested themselves in more popular works. *One Flew Over the Cuckoo's Nest* (1962), Ken Kesey's novel depicting a ward's tyrannical regime, captured a wide public both as a best-seller and as a movie.

Fighting for Human Rights

I NSPIRED by the successes black citizens had during the 1960s in getting federal courts to guarantee and expand their rights, lawyers filed a number of important suits on behalf of mentally ill people, starting in the late 1960s. The most important cases have involved commitment procedures, the rights of patients in central institutions, the right to care in the least restrictive setting possible, securing services and benefits in the community and barring discrimination against mentally ill people in the job market, education and housing.

In the landmark case of *Wyatt v. Stickney,* U.S. District Judge Frank M. Johnson handed down a decision in April 1972 ordering the Alabama state government to maintain specified minimum standards in all state institutions. Judge Johnson said every mentally impaired person should be assured the right to the least restrictive setting possible, and he ordered the state to set up "human rights committees" for each institution.

As the result of another significant 1972 decision, *Lessard v. Schmidt,* the state of Wisconsin was required to review 7,000 cases of involuntarily committed persons, on grounds that commitment procedures had violated constitutional guarantees of due process. Three years later, the U.S. Supreme Court ruled in *O'Conner v. Donaldson* (1975) that patients "who are not dangerous to themselves or others, are receiving only custodial care and are capable of surviving safely in freedom or with the help of family or friends" could not be institutionalized against their will.[33] In *Addington v. Texas* (1979), the Supreme Court held that the need for a person to be confined in a mental institution had to be demonstrated by "clear and convincing" evidence rather than by a mere "preponderance of evidence." [34]

A federal law enacted in 1980 authorized the Justice Department to bring suits against states on behalf of people confined to institutions.[35] Generally, though, the Supreme Court has

[33] 422 U.S. 563 (1975).
[34] 441 U.S. 418 (1979).
[35] See Congressional Quarterly's *Almanac* (1980), pp. 383-384.

been extremely reluctant to entertain the notion that mentally ill people have a constitutional right to some specific level of treatment. This June, for the first time, the court handed down a decision that seems to guarantee a minimum right to treatment for the institutionalized mentally ill.

The case, *Younger v. Romeo,* involved a retarded man who had been injured some 70 times as an inmate at Pennsylvania's Pennhurst State School. By an 8-1 majority, the court ruled that inmates in such institutions have a right to at least enough training to assure their physical safety and a reasonable amount of freedom. Writing for the majority, Justice Lewis F. Powell Jr. said that "persons who have been involuntarily committed are entitled to more considerate treatment and conditions of confinement than criminals whose conditions of confinement are designed to punish." [36]

Justice Powell emphasized in his decision that "courts must show deference to the judgment exercised by qualified professionals" in assessing institutional services, since "there certainly is no reason to think judges or juries are better qualified than appropriate professionals in making such decisions." In issuing this warning, Powell sought to rein in activist judges who might otherwise inject themselves too much into the technicalities of managing institutions.

However, in the estimation of Norman Rosenberg, director of the Mental Health Law Project in Washington, judges have been more restrained than commonly thought. It is partly for this reason, Rosenberg said, that many more suits have been brought on behalf of retarded people in state facilities than on behalf of the institutionalized mentally ill. In many institutions for the retarded, Rosenberg explained, essentially nothing was being done for inmates, and so it was relatively easy to persuade courts that residents deserved some kind of professional treatment; in mental institutions, on the other hand, patients usually receive some professional care, and in these cases it is much harder to get judges to make technical judgments about how much care is enough.[37]

Rosenberg said that it has been even harder to bring suits on behalf of mentally ill people in the community. When the state confines a sick or disabled person, the principle is well established in law that the state assumes some reciprocal responsibilities toward the person. When the person is discharged into the community, however, the state has no special responsibilities under constitutional or common law toward the individual.

---

[36] Last year, in another decision involving Pennhurst, the Supreme Court ruled that a 1975 federal law did not by itself require states to provide retarded people with a specific level of treatment. See "Changes in Mental Retardation Care," *E.R.R.*, 1982 Vol. I, p. 464.
[37] Interview, June 24, 1982.

Because of this, Rosenberg said, legal advocates for mentally ill people often find themselves in a "Catch-22 situation." While they may be able to secure the release of patients from institutions, there is often little they can do for the patients once they are in the community.

To date, only a couple of suits have resulted in courts ordering the establishment of more adequate community care. In the Dixon case, in which the Mental Health Law Project has been deeply involved, U.S. District Court Judge Aubrey Robinson handed down a decision in December 1975 that held the District of Columbia and federal governments jointly responsible for providing outpatient care in the community for people discharged from St. Elizabeths Hospital.[38] According to press reports, the two governments did not meet that responsibility with any great dispatch, and in a consent decree approved by the court on April 30, 1980, they were obligated to provide specified services by specified dates. The order provides for establishment of a plaintiffs' monitoring committee to review implementation of the plan over a five-year period.

In *Brewster v. Dukakis,* a suit filed against the Massachusetts state government in 1976, a 1978 consent degree required the establishment of community services for people discharged from institutions in western Massachusetts. Steven Schwartz, director of the Mental Patients' Advocacy Project in Northampton, Mass., said there has been "a pretty dramatic increase" in services since 1978, though not as great as the decree called for.[39]

Advocacy Groups; Problem of Stigmatization

Efforts have been unavailing to get Congress to spell out in law the rights that states should guarantee the mentally ill. The 1975 Developmental Disabilities Act contained a national bill of rights for the retarded and other handicapped people, but proposals to include a comparable statement in the 1980 Mental Health Systems Act encountered stiff opposition. Congress ended up merely recommending a model bill of rights for adoption by state legislatures.

Groups representing the mentally ill apparently have not organized as effectively in recent decades as groups speaking for the retarded. The National Mental Health Association, the descendant of an organization that was founded in 1909, currently has about 8,000 dues-paying members and 850 local

[38] See Mental Health Law Project, "Summary of Activities: July 1979-June 1981," pp. 6-7. The Mental Health Law Project was founded in 1972, in response to Judge Johnson's ruling in *Wyatt v. Stickney,* by representatives of the Center for Law and Social Policy, the American Civil Liberties Union and the American Orthopsychiatric Association. It acts as a legal advocacy group for mentally ill and mentally retarded people.
[39] Interview, July 16, 1982.

chapters in 45 states.[40] The Association for Retarded Citizens, by comparison, has a membership of about 200,000 and affiliates in 48 states. About half of ARC's membership consists of parents or siblings of retarded people, while the Mental Health Association's membership is a more diffuse mixture of concerned citizens and health-care personnel.

In an attempt to emulate ARC, 250 people met in Madison, Wis., in September 1979 to found the National Alliance for the Mentally Ill. It has 126 affiliates in all parts of the country and focuses mainly on the problems of chronic mental patients and it stresses the need for more neurobiological research as the key to helping such people. It shares many positions with the Mental Health Association, but its officers believe that the association takes too broad a view of mental health and devotes too much attention to the problems of the "worried well."

All advocates for the mentally ill complain about the stigmatization that the afflicted continue to suffer from. While mentally retarded people are increasingly regarded as victims of circumstances, there is a lingering notion, not easily dispelled, that mentally disturbed people are somehow responsible for their condition. Since it is often hard to distinguish the insane from the healthy, there is understandably a feeling that people acting crazy ought to be able to improve their condition if they just tried harder — and sometimes, it seems, they can.

There is also a fear, not completely unfounded, that mental illness is somewhat contagious — that emotionally disturbed people will drive their families and friends crazy, if given the chance.[41] On top of that, it is widely believed that most mentally ill people are violent. Specialists say that mentally ill people do not commit crimes any more frequently than normal individuals from comparable economic and social backgrounds, but sound, comprehensive studies seem to be lacking, and sensational stories about crimes committed by deranged people appear often and attract wide attention. A recent study by two professors at Vanderbilt University found that a surprisingly large number of elderly mental patients commit violent acts.[42]

Insanity and Criminality; Hinckley Backlash

The recent federal court trial of John W. Hinckley Jr., who shot President Reagan and three others on March 30, 1981, focused national attention on some of the sticky issues that come up when the law encounters psychiatry. The trial was a

[40] Its ancestor, the National Committee for Mental Hygiene, was founded in 1909 by Clifford W. Beers, a former mental patient who described his experiences in a best-selling book, *A Mind that Found Itself* (1908).
[41] Parents of mentally ill people are reported to have a divorce rate of about 50 percent. See Johnson, *op. cit.*, p. 18.
[42] See *Journal of the American Medical Association*, July 23.

reminder that professional psychiatrists and psychologists still are unable to agree about something as basic as who is sane and who is insane. The jury's verdict, in which Hinckley was found not guilty by reason of insanity, ran counter to the testimony of some of the psychiatrists and met with public skepticism and outright hostility. In its wake have come calls for elimination of the insanity defense or its modification to read "guilty but insane."

Increasingly, psychiatrists and mental health program directors are finding themselves bearing the brunt of public outrage when mental patients or former mental patients commit crimes. In a California case, a crime victim's family brought a malpractice suit successfully against a psychiatrist who took no preventive action after a patient told him of his intention to commit a crime. In other cases, psychiatrists connected with institutions have come under fire for releasing patients with criminal records who commit new crimes after their discharge.

Harry Schnibbe, director of the National Association of State Mental Health Program Directors, said forensic psychiatry has become the leading issue affecting his constituency.[43] Schnibbe said that mental health directors are in court "all the time now" for one reason or another. Either they are defending their systems against charges that they abuse human rights, Schnibbe said, or they are up against complaints about releasing criminally violent people into the community. Schnibbe's organization includes a division of forensic directors and a division of state legal counsels.

Rosenberg, director of the Mental Health Law Project, said that Schnibbe's concerns are reminiscent of age-old fears about "lawyers taking over the world." Rosenberg asserted that there have been, in fact, very few successful suits brought against mental health care personnel for dealing carelessly with the criminally insane. He agreed with other specialists in the field that mentally ill people are not abnormally inclined to commit crimes, though he knew of no readily available studies that could be used to document this claim in meetings with concerned citizens. Until there are authoritative data on the issues raised by cases like Hinckley's, it seems improbable that communities will feel altogether at ease about providing homes for discharged mental patients.

---

[43] Interview, June 18, 1982.

Selected Bibliography

Books

Ennis, Bruce J. and Richard D. Emery, *The Rights of Mental Patients: The Revised Edition of the Basic American Civil Liberties Guide to a Mental Patient's Rights*, Avon, 1978.

Halpern, Joseph and others, *The Myths of Deinstitutionalization: Policies for the Mentally Disabled*, Westview Press, 1980.

Rubin, Jeffrey, *Economics, Mental Health and the Law*, D. C. Heath and Co., 1978.

Sheehan, Susan, *Is There No Place on Earth for Me?* Houghton Mifflin Co., 1982.

Articles

Bachrach, Leona L., "A Conceptual Approach to Deinstitutionalization," *Hospital and Community Psychiatry*, September 1978.

Bassuk, Ellen L. and Samuel Gerson, "Deinstitutionalization and Mental Health Services," *Scientific American*, February 1978.

Hatfield, Agnes B., "Self-Help Groups for Families of the Mentally Ill," *Social Work*, September 1981.

___ "The Family as Partner in the Treatment of Mental Illness," *Hospital and Community Psychiatry*, Sept. 9, 1981.

Lamb, H. Richard, "Securing Patients' Rights — Responsibly," *Hospital and Community Psychiatry*, June 1981.

Smith, W. G. and Donald W. Hart, "Community Mental Health: A Noble Failure?" *Hospital and Community Psychiatry*, September 1975.

Winslow, Walter W., "Changing Trends in Community Health Centers," *Hospital and Community Psychiatry*, April 1982.

Reports and Studies

American Federation of State, County and Municipal Employees, "Patients for Sale: How Private Profit Exploits the Mentally Disabled," Washington, 1980.

___ Special reports on placement of the mentally ill and retarded in Florida, Minnesota, Missouri and Illinois, all dated 1980.

Editorial Research Reports: "Changes in Mental Retardation Care," 1982 Vol. I, p. 449; "Mental Health Care," 1979 Vol. II, p. 681; "Brain Research," 1978 Vol. I, p. 61; "Psychomedicine," 1974 Vol. I, p. 497; "Schizophrenia, Medical Enigma," 1972 Vol. I, p. 233.

General Accounting Office, "Returning the Mentally Disabled to the Community: Government Needs to Do More," Washington, Jan. 7, 1977.

National Institute of Mental Health, Survey and Reports Branch, "Provisional Data on Federally Funded Community Mental Health Centers, 1978-79," Washington, September 1981.

The President's Commission on Mental Health, "Report to the President," Washington, 1978.

___ "Report of the Task Panel on Deinstitutionalization, Rehabilitation and Long-Term Care," Feb. 15, 1978.

Santiestevan, Henry, "Deinstitutionalization: Out of Their Beds and Into the Streets," AFSCME, Washington, December 1976.

NEW CANCER TREATMENTS

by

Marc Leepson

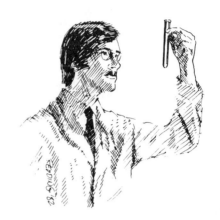

**Jan. 29
1 9 8 2**

NEW CANCER TREATMENTS

W HEN BILLIONAIRE industrialist Armand Hammer talks, people listen. Hammer, chairman of Occidental Petroleum Corp., recently donated $2 million in prizes and awards to the fight against cancer, including $1 million to any scientist who finds a cure for cancer by 1991.[1] Hammer's offer provides a sharp illustration of the nation's continuing concern with cancer — a disease that kills some 420,000 Americans a year. Even though survival rates for most cancers have improved in recent years, cancer remains one of the most feared maladies. Most cancers bring intense pain and suffering for the patient, and anxiety and uncertainty for family and friends.

Doctors still do not know what causes the disease or precisely why some treatments are successful and others are not. What is certain is that one in four living Americans will contract cancer in their lifetime, that cancer strikes about two of every three families, and that about 800,000 new cancer patients were diagnosed in 1981.[2] Medical researchers have linked cigarette smoking with most cases of lung cancer, frequent overexposure to direct sunlight with most skin cancers, and exposure to industrial chemicals such as asbestos with other types of cancer. But the exact causes of most cancers remain a medical mystery.

There are some 10 billion cells in the average adult body. Cancer begins when a single cell undergoes an abnormal change and starts to spread uncontrollably. Groups of runaway cancer cells grow into masses of tissue called tumors (see glossary, p. 104). Benign tumors do not spread throughout the body. Malignant tumors do expand; they invade and destroy normal body tissues. Most cancers stay at their original site for a period of time, when they are known as localized cancers. Eventually, most cancers move into organs and tissues, or become detached and course through the lymph or blood systems to other parts of the body. This process is called metastasis. When cancer cells metastasize throughout the entire body, they cause death.

The good news about cancer is the increasing effectiveness of today's treatment techniques, which for the most part involve

---

[1] Hammer, who is head of President Reagan's cancer advisory panel, made the offer on Dec. 3, 1981.
[2] Statistics from American Cancer Society, "Cancer Facts and Figures, 1982."

Glossary of Cancer Terms

Cancer. A general term, derived from the Latin word meaning crab, used to indicate any of various types of malignant diseases that invade the body and are likely to result in illness or death.

Carcinogen. A term used to describe any cancer-producing agent.

Carcinoma. A solid malignant tumor that originates in the skin, glands, nerves, breasts, lungs, stomach, digestive and urinary tracts. Carcinoma accounts for 80 to 90 percent of all cancer cases in the United States.

Leukemia. Cancer of the blood-producing organs caused by the overproduction of immature white corpuscles; it accounts for about 4 percent of all U.S. cancer cases.

Lymphoma. A form of cancer resulting from an abnormal production of immature lymphocytes by the spleen and lymph nodes; **Hodgkin's disease**, the most common type of lymphoma, accounts for about 3 percent of all cancers.

Melanoma. A fast-growing malignant tumor.

Sarcoma. A solid malignant tumor growing in muscle, bone, cartilage and connective tissue; it accounts for only about 2 percent of the U.S. cancer cases.

Tumor. A mass of abnormal tissue arising from pre-existing cells, serving no known purpose and growing independently of surrounding tissue. Benign tumors cause damage only when they interfere with the function of an organ. Malignant tumors kill by causing generalized emaciation and ill health in the host. They do not produce toxins, but take a priority on the body's nutrients, ultimately causing infections and organ failures.

combinations of surgery, radiation and chemotherapy. Survival rates for cancer patients are higher than ever before. ". . . Forty-five percent of the 785,000 patients diagnosed with serious cancers in 1980 are curable," said Dr. Vincent T. DeVita Jr., director of the National Cancer Institute. "These curable patients include 219,850 with localized disease who are curable by surgery alone; approximately 90,000 patients curable as a result of radiation and surgery; and 46,000 curable as a result of using chemotherapy alone or with surgery and/or radiation therapy. None of the figures include early skin or cervical cancers, which are nearly 100 percent curable." [3]

Recent Advances in Fight Against Cancer

Some of the biggest advances have come in treating childhood cancers. Cancer is relatively rare in children — only about 6,200 young people were diagnosed with cancer in this country last year. Nevertheless, cancer is the chief cause of death by disease of those aged 3 to 14; about 2,300 children died from cancer in 1981. Malignancies develop more rapidly in young persons than

[3] Quoted in "Cancer Patient Survival: An Update," National Cancer Institute, Nov. 30, 1981.

in adults. This is because children's bodies grow rapidly and cancer tends to grow with them. The most common childhood cancers are leukemia — which accounted for about half the childhood cancer deaths last year — and cancers of the bone, brain, nervous system and kidneys.

The five-year survival rates[4] for most children's cancers have grown markedly in the last 10 years. A decade ago a child stricken with acute lymphotic leukemia (the most common childhood cancer) had only a 25-to-30 percent chance of living five years. Today, 50-to-75 percent of childhood leukemia victims survive at least that long. The success of treating childhood cancers prompted a highly optimistic forecast from one childhood cancer specialist. "I believe we can look forward to curing childhood cancer in our lifetime," said Dr. Michael Harris, chief of pediatric hematology and oncology at the Mt. Sinai Medical Center in New York.[5]

Increases in the Five-Year Survival Rates

Along with the increasing survival rates in children's cancers has come equally promising improvements in the survival rates for most other forms of the disease. A five-year study conducted by the American College of Surgeons released in September 1981 analyzed treatments and results of 468,288 cancer patients whose diseases were diagnosed after 1972. The results were compared with data from a similar survey conducted by the National Cancer Institute (NCI) from 1965-69. The College of Surgeons' survey found that the survival rates for patients with many common cancers have risen significantly. Some 73 percent of those diagnosed with breast cancer after 1972 survived for at least five years, compared to 65 percent of those diagnosed in the earlier period. The surival rate for cancer of the colon rose from 46 to 50 percent; for prostate cancer, from 57 to 68 percent; uterine cancer, from 75 to 84 percent; and Hodgkin's disease, from 54 to 72 percent. "The results of the new study indicate we are making good strides against common cancers and excellent progress against the rarer ones," said Dr. Charles Smart, director of the cancer department of the American College of Surgeons and a clinical professor of surgery at the University of Utah.[6]

The preliminary results of a new NCI study generally support the findings of the American College of Surgeons. The NCI survey, released Nov. 30, 1981, found that about 45 percent of those diagnosed with serious cancers in 1973 and 1974 survived

---

[4] Doctors usually consider cancer "cured" if a patient survives for five years after the cancer is diagnosed. The National Cancer Institute studied cancer patients whose diseases were diagnosed from 1950-54, and found that 85 percent of those who had survived for five years lived for at least 20 years.

[5] Quoted in *Harper's Bazaar*, December 1981, p. 209.

[6] See *The Bulletin of the American College of Surgeons*, September 1981, pp. 5-13.

for five years, compared to a 40 percent five-year survival rate for those diagnosed with cancer from 1967 to 1973. NCI researchers point out that the new and old data are not strictly comparable because the earlier statistics came primarily from patients in teaching hospitals affiliated with universities, while the new data was supplied by the institute's SEER (Surveillance, Epidemiology and End Results) program using statistics from a 10 percent sample of the hospital population.[7] Nevertheless, the survey results indicate that cancer patients are "living longer than ever before," Dr. DeVita said.

NCI officials and others involved in cancer research and treatment say that cancer patients now have a greater chance of survival for two basic reasons: the growing tendency among patients and doctors to detect cancers earlier and the marked advances in chemotherapy in the last decade. Chemotherapy, a treatment involving the use of drugs in large doses, cannot help all cancer patients. Chemotherapy usually is most effective in fighting cancers in otherwise healthy patients whose cancers are in their early, localized stages.

One problem with chemotherapy is that most anti-cancer drugs attack both cancer cells and normal, healthy ones. In doing so, these powerful drugs usually cause unwanted side effects, ranging from nausea to, in extreme cases, death. "The same drugs that destroy [cancer] cells also destroy white blood cells, hair cells and other fast-growing cells. This destruction is responsible for the hair loss, nausea, fatigue and susceptibility to other diseases, which, for some patients have made these cures more painful than the cancer," wrote journalist Andrew Silk, a recovering lung cancer patient. "In a paradox typical of current cancer treatment, my survival depended largely on how much poison I could withstand."[8] According to chemotherapy critic Ralph W. Moss, "All of these drugs have one characteristic in common. They are all poisonous. They work because they're poisons."[9]

Debate Over Use of Experimental Drugs

Chemotherapy's side effects are very taxing for patients receiving proven cancer treatments. But chemotherapy causes an extra burden for those who take unproven, experimental drugs. These patients, nearly all of whom have little chance for survival, get the tortuous side effects without any assurance

---

[7] The SEER program, which began in 1972, is run by the institute's Biometry Branch. SEER statistics are gleaned from 11 areas of the country: parts of Michigan, Georgia, Louisiana, Washington, California, the entire states of Connecticut, Iowa, New Mexico, Utah and Hawaii and the entire Commonwealth of Puerto Rico. The statistics measure cancer incidence and mortality and are classified according to sex, race, age, residence of the patient, site and type of cancer.

[8] Writing in *The New York Times Magazine*, Oct. 18, 1981, p. 36.

[9] Ralph W. Moss, *The Cancer Syndrome* (1980), p. 62.

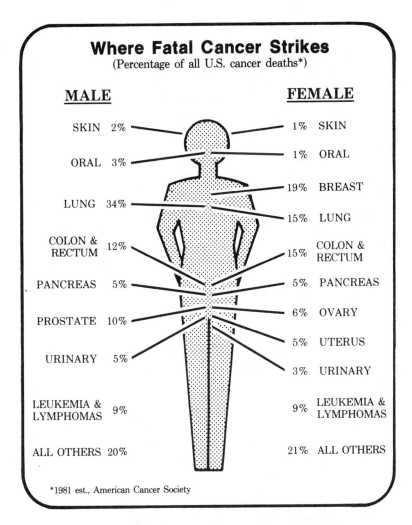

Where Fatal Cancer Strikes
(Percentage of all U.S. cancer deaths*)

MALE   FEMALE

MALE			FEMALE
SKIN	2%	1%	SKIN
ORAL	3%	1%	ORAL
		19%	BREAST
LUNG	34%	15%	LUNG
COLON & RECTUM	12%	15%	COLON & RECTUM
PANCREAS	5%	5%	PANCREAS
		6%	OVARY
PROSTATE	10%	5%	UTERUS
URINARY	5%	3%	URINARY
LEUKEMIA & LYMPHOMAS	9%	9%	LEUKEMIA & LYMPHOMAS
ALL OTHERS	20%	21%	ALL OTHERS

*1981 est., American Cancer Society

that the drugs will help them. There is an ongoing debate over the use of experimental drugs on terminal cancer patients. The argument intensified last October following publication of a four-part series of articles in *The Washington Post* that sharply criticized the cancer establishment in general and the National Cancer Institute in particular for the widespread use of experimental drugs on cancer patients.

Reporters Ted Gup and Jonathan Newmann, who researched the issue for 12 months, found 620 cases in which experimental drugs were "implicated" in the deaths of cancer patients. Those deaths, the reporters wrote, "amounted to merely a fraction of the thousands of people who in recent years have died or suffered terribly from cancer experiments...." [10]

[10] Writing in *The Washington Post*, Oct. 18, 1981. The series ran on Oct. 18, 19, 20 and 21.

Gup and Newmann said that since 1971 more than 150 experimental drugs have been given in NCI-sponsored tests to tens of thousands of patients. As is the case with proven anti-cancer drugs, many of the experimental substances were derived from highly toxic industrial chemicals such as pesticides, herbicides and dyes. Cancer researchers use these drugs on terminally ill patients after the drugs show positive results in laboratory animals. Gup and Newmann claimed that some of the experimental drugs were carcinogenic (cancer causing), that some of the experiments' results contained misleading and falsified information and that some drugs were given to patients without having been approved by the Food and Drug Administration. "The litany of death and suffering from experimental drugs has become an accepted part of life at some hospitals," the reporters said. "These human experiments have gone largely unchallenged and unquestioned by Congress, the medical profession and the scientific community at large."

The articles brought immediate and critical response from cancer researchers involved in testing experimental drugs. Vincent DeVita of the National Cancer Institute said the reporters showed a "tragic lack of understanding of cancer treatment and the national program to develop drugs that are effective in treating cancer" and a "slanted and distorted view of cancer research." DeVita said that cancer patients and doctors are interested only in treating cancer, not in experimenting with drugs. "In this context, many patients feel that it is worthwhile putting up with side effects of treatment knowing that the treatment may prolong their lives or provide a cure," he said. "The possibility of treatment side effects and the small but real chance of drug-related death has to be balanced against the nearly 100 percent chance of death if experimental therapy is not attempted on the advanced cancer patients who participate in our studies." [11]

Dr. James F. Holland, director of the cancer department at Mt. Sinai Medical Center in New York City, also criticized the newspaper's allegations. Holland characterized the articles as a "lopsided view of an intellectual pursuit of great importance to humanity ... entirely without balance in terms of the benefits to be recognized from experimental drug treatments, and ... done as if these were poisons and not drugs on the way to potential therapeutic application." [12]

Dr. Robert Benjamin, chief of clinical pharmacology at the University of Texas' M. D. Anderson Hospital and Tumor Institute in Houston, whose experimental program was criticized

---

[11] Statement published in *The Washington Post*, Oct. 19, 1981.
[12] Appearing on "The MacNeil/Lehrer Report," PBS-TV, Oct. 26, 1981.

in the *Post* series, also spoke out recently on the subject. Benjamin said that chemotherapy must be viewed in perspective. "Experimental cancer drugs are only given to patients with their consent when death is imminent and every known therapy has been exhausted," he said. "An experimental drug's risk of causing toxic side effects must be balanced against the patient's certain death." Dr. Gerald P. Bodey Sr. of M. D. Anderson Hospital added: "We would love to have drugs that are nontoxic, but cancer cells are not too dissimilar from normal human cells. So it's very hard to find something that's going to have an effect on cancer cells and not on normal cells." [13]

"The possibility of treatment side effects and the small but real chance of drug-related death has to be balanced against the nearly 100 percent chance of death if experimental therapy is not attempted on the advanced cancer patients who participate in our studies."

Dr. Vincent T. DeVita Jr.
Director of the National Cancer Institute

The newspaper articles prompted a congressional hearing on the subject of experimental drugs. Rep. Henry A. Waxman, D-Calif., said at the Oct. 27, 1981, hearing that some cancer patients do not know that "they are being used as guinea pigs to see how much toxic effect a drug will have and that any value to them is remote." [14] Dr. DeVita defended his agency's experimental program, testifying that only about 3 percent of the 1,400 cancer patients who took Phase I, or preliminary, chemotherapy treatments in the previous 18 months had died from the experimental drugs, while about 9.5 percent of those in the experimental program were helped by the new drugs. New drugs "are tested first on people who desperately need help," he said. "Fully 90 percent of patients in Phase I trials fail to respond to a drug and die within a year."

The Investigations and Oversight Subcommittee of the Senate Labor and Human Resources Committee also held a hearing on the subject Nov. 3. The panel, chaired by Sen. Paula Hawkins, R-Fla., had been investigating NCI's drug program since early in 1981. Speaking on the Senate floor Oct. 19, 1981, Sen.

---

[13] Drs. Benjamin and Bodey were interviewed in Houston by Editorial Research Reports contributor Sari Horwitz.
[14] The hearing was sponsored jointly by the Health Subcommittee of the House Energy and Commerce Committee and the Investigations Subcommittee of the House Science and Technology Committee.

Hawkins said the subcommittee had uncovered "serious deficiencies" in NCI's drug development program and the Food and Drug Administration's regulation of new anti-cancer drugs. Hawkins said the "most serious problem" was "the lack of an adequate program for monitoring hundreds of NCI-sponsored human experiments involving 95 new anti-cancer drugs."

Search for Cancer Cures

CANCER has been known and feared since ancient times. Evidence of the disease has been found in fossil bones, and there are descriptions of cancer symptoms in Egyptian papyri.[15] The 4th century B.C. Greek physician Hippocrates, considered the father of medicine, studied the disease and coined the term "carcinoma" for what we know as the solid malignant tumor that accounts for 80 to 90 percent of all cancer cases. Hippocrates, who believed that cancer was caused by an excess of black bile, recommended not treating cancerous tumors. "If treated, the patients die quickly," he wrote, "but if not treated, they hold out for a long time."[16] The Latin encyclopediast Celsus, who wrote a medical encyclopedia in the first century A.D., saw no hope in treating advanced cancers. Celsus believed that the rudimentary surgical techniques of his age were too dangerous.

The attack on cancer by modern scientific methods dates from the 18th century. The world's first cancer hospital was set up in Rheims, France, in the mid-1700s, but it was soon closed when fears grew in the surrounding area that cancer was contagious. Later in that century cancer hospitals were established in England and the United States, among them New York Cancer Hospital, which later became the Memorial Sloan-Kettering Cancer Center, and Roswell Park Memorial Institute in Buffalo. Other leading American cancer research centers are the M. D. Anderson Hospital and Tumor Clinic in Houston and the Sidney Farber Cancer Institute in Boston.

Improvements in Radiation Treatments

Nearly 90 percent of all cancer cases in this country involve tumors. In most cases the first step in treating malignant tumors is surgical removal. If the cancer is in the preliminary, localized state, surgery usually wipes out the disease. If the tumor is not excised completely, surgery is augmented with radiation and/or chemotherapy.

---

[15] See "Quest for Cancer Control," *E.R.R.*, 1974 Vol. II, pp. 623-641.
[16] See Michael B. Shimkin, "Contrary to Nature," an account of cancer history published by the National Institutes of Health in 1977.

Doctors began experimenting with radiation as a cancer treatment soon after radium was discovered in the late 1890s. Radiation is effective against cancer cells because they tend to be more sensitive than normal cells to radiation's toxic effects. Certain cancers, including those that affect the lymph nodes, often respond favorably to radiation therapy. Other cancers are very resistant. In some cases, such as localized cancers of the prostate and larynx, radiation is used instead of surgery. Unlike surgery, radiation does not disfigure or harm non-effected organs.

Cancer researchers are continually searching for ways to improve radiation therapy. One new experimental technique uses implanted radioactive pellets that deliver radiation into the body. Doctors believe they may be able to pinpoint the pellets to reach cancer cells without harming normal cells. Radiologists also are working with drugs called radiosensitizers that are injected into the body and attach themselves to cancer cells. These drugs also help the radiation zero in on the cancer cells.

Like chemotherapy, radiation can cause unwanted side-effects such as nausea, vomiting and loss of appetite. There is the additional possibility that radiation itself may cause cancer.[17] Journalist Andrew Silk, who received radiation for small-cell carcinoma of the lung (also known as oat-cell cancer), said: "Although the treatment was painless, I grew increasingly tired, my throat was sore and I lost much of my appetite."

Chemotherapy Successful in Some Cases

Chemotherapy dates from 1865 when doctors began giving doses of arsenic to leukemia patients. Little progress was made for decades. Then during World War II a team of researchers working with chemical-warfare compounds at Yale University discovered that nitrogen mustard, a relative of the deadly mustard gas, killed cancer cells. After animal tests, researchers administered the drug to a patient with lymphosarcoma, a fast-spreading cancer. The nitrogen mustard inhibited the cancer's growth. Nitrogen mustard was approved for medical use as a treatment for lymph cancer and Hodgkin's disease, the most common type of lymphoma, in 1948.

With that promising beginning, scientists began searching for other drugs that would combat cancer. The search was — and remains — a hit-and-miss process. Many of the drugs that have proven to be effective were discovered by happenstance. The National Cancer Institute, which had been set up in 1937, began a program in 1955 to help researchers find reliable cancer-fighting drugs. Since then, hundreds of millions of dollars have

---

[17] See "Determining Radiation Dangers," *E.R.R.*, 1979 Vol. II, pp. 561-580.

been spent on the effort. NCI's current yearly budget for drug development now exceeds $50 million. It is estimated that about $1 billion a year is spent in this country on cancer research by both government and private groups.

There are at least 50 different drugs that have had some success in fighting cancer. Oncologists (cancer specialists) often use combinations of drugs in fighting cancers. Combination chemotherapy usually minimizes side effects because each drug is given in moderate doses. Dr. DeVita of the National Cancer Institute estimates that as many as 46,000 cancer patients are cured every year in this country with chemotherapy — about 6 percent of the approximately 805,000 cancer cases diagnosed annually. Chemotherapy is most successful with the following cancers:

Acute lymphotic leukemia. One of the main types of leukemia, this disease hits the lymphocytes, which are produced in the lymph nodes and bone marrow. Acute lymphotic leukemia occurs most frequently in children. Until relatively recently, children contracting this disease rarely survived more than a few months. But now 50-to-75 percent of children who contract acute lymphotic leukemia live for five years and are considered cured; about 90 percent receive some form of temporary relief, called remission. The drugs used to treat acute lymphotic leukemia include asparaginase, mercaptopurine, methotrexate, prednisone, thioguanine and vincristine sulfate.

Hodgkin's disease. A cancer of the lymph glands that usually affects young adults and children. In the last decade doctors have had great success in treating this disease. According to NCI statistics, 90 percent of the children who contracted Hodgkin's disease in the early 1970s have been cured, along with 69 percent of the female adults and 66 percent of the male adults. Among the drugs used to combat Hodgkin's disease are lomustine, prednisone, procarbazine, vinblastine and vincristine sulfates.

Choriocarcinoma. A cancer of the placenta that affects pregnant women, this disease is cured in about 70 percent of cases with a combination of methotrexate, dactinomycin and vinblastine.

Testicular cancer in males and **ovarian cancer** in females both respond very favorably to cisplatin, a compound derived from platinum that is one of the most widely used anti-cancer drugs. Used in combination with surgery, cisplatin now cures about 85 percent of all testicular cancer cases and about 40 percent of ovarian cancers.

Other cancers that have responded favorably to chemotherapy are: Wilms' tumor, a kidney cancer in children; Ewing's sarcoma, a bone tumor; Burkitt's lymphoma, a malignant lymphoma found primarily in African children and only rarely in the United States; embryonal rhabdomyosarcoma, a malignant muscle cancer; and osteogenic sarcoma, the most common malignant bone sarcoma that usually affects the ends of long bones and is found usually in those aged 10-25.

These are relatively rare cancers. As for some of the most common cancers, NCI statistics on five-year survival are not as encouraging. Lung cancer, for example, has proven to be all but immune to chemotherapy. Lung cancer accounts for about 20 percent of all cancer deaths; about 100,000 Americans died of that disease in 1981. The five-year survival rate for lung cancer cases diagnosed from 1970-73 is only 10 percent for whites and 7 percent for blacks, according to the latest NCI statistics. Cancer of the colon and rectum accounted for 13.6 percent of all cancer deaths in 1981, second only to lung cancer. The five-year survival rates for those and other leading cancers follow:

Type of Cancer		Five-Year Survival Rates for Cases Diagnosed in	
		1960-63	1970-73
colon	whites	43%	49%
	blacks	34	37
rectum	whites	38	45
	blacks	28	30
breast	whites	63	68
	blacks	46	51
prostate	whites	50	63
	blacks	35	55
bladder	whites	53	61
	blacks	24	35
uterus (other than cervix)	whites	73	81
	blacks	31	44
pancreas	whites	1	1
	blacks	1	2
cervix	whites	58	64
	blacks	47	61
stomach	whites	11	13
	blacks	8	13

Cancer researchers say the differences between black and white survival rates owe more to environmental and socio-economic factors than to genetic characteristics. "Because a higher percentage of blacks than whites are in the lower socio-economic group, risk of exposure to industrial carcinogens may be increased," the American Cancer Society reported. "Also, limited educational opportunities may prevent early detection as the less educated are less likely to know the importance of symptoms which could lead to an early diagnosis." [18]

[18] American Cancer Society, "Cancer Facts and Figures, 1982," p. 5.

Promising New Treatments

THE GENERAL, accepted medical treatments for cancer today are surgery, radiation and chemotherapy. But medical practitioners also offer dozens of other cancer treatments, from positive thinking and biofeedback to massive doses of Vitamin C or the industrial solvent DMSO. Researchers also are working on pioneering methods of fighting cancer, including several different types of immunotherapy treatments in which doctors induce substances into cancer patients' bodies that help the body's own disease defenses counteract cancer cells. Interferon, a substance naturally produced in the body in response to viral infections, is being closely examined as a potential cancer cure. Hyperthermia, an ancient cancer-fighting method that subjects patients to heat therapy, has been proven effective in fighting certain cancers, including skin cancer.

It is easy to understand why cancer patients and their families turn to experimental therapies. Dying of cancer is one of life's most painful and distressing experiences. It can involve months of agonizing physical and mental pain. Conventional medicine in many cases offers little or no chance for relief or cure. In anger and frustration cancer patients sometimes opt for unproven treatments.

A case in point involves Laetrile, a drug that gained notoriety in the early 1970s as a so-called cancer miracle drug. The Food and Drug Administration in 1975 declared Laetrile "worthless" as a cancer cure; the American Cancer Society characterized the drug in 1973 as "quackery." [19] Laetrile is a trade-name for amygdalin, a carbohydrate found in plants including wild cherry bark, sorghum and apricot pits. After the FDA banned the sale and interstate shipment of Laetrile, proponents of patients' rights to choose their own cancer-fighting treatments formed activist groups advocating "freedom of choice." Intense lobbying resulted in the passage by 23 state legislatures of laws legalizing the drug. In other states courts have allowed some patients to receive Laetrile from their doctors.

The Supreme Court, which in 1979 had ruled that FDA could legally stop the distribution of Laetrile, last year declined to review a challenge to the FDA ban. Results of the most recent NCI-sponsored Laetrile tests, released April 30, 1981, show that none of 156 cancer patients studied were helped by the drug in a nine-month period. Some of the participants were also put on a diet that emphasized fresh fruit, vegetables and whole grains,

---

[19] See Terri Schultz and Bard Lindeman, "The Victimization of Desperate Cancer Patients," *Today's Health,* November 1973.

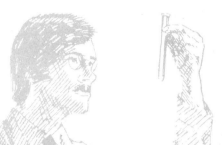

In 1982 about 835,000 Americans will be diagnosed as having cancer and about 430,000 will die of the disease.

Of every five deaths in the United States, one is from cancer.

Cancer is the chief cause of death by disease of those aged 3 to 14; about 2,300 children died from cancer in 1981.

About 45 percent of the patients diagnosed with serious cancers today are curable, compared to about 40 percent a decade ago.

and restricted animal products, salt, alcohol and refined sugar. Laetrile proponents charged that the NCI study was not accurately compiled, and dismissed the negative evidence as another medical establishment attempt to dismiss Laetile's effectiveness.

Experiments with Chemical Solvent DMSO

A similar controversy is brewing over the use of dimethyl sulfoxide (DMSO), a chemical solvent that is a byproduct of papermaking. DMSO is widely prescribed in Europe, Canada and Australia to heal sores and bruises and reduce the pain associated with cancer. In this country the FDA has approved DMSO for use in treating one type of bladder condition, and has sanctioned DMSO experiments. The National Cancer Institute is testing DMSO as a cancer treatment at the Baltimore Cancer Research Center. The substance being tested by NCI contains 50 percent DMSO; but the DMSO usually sold in this country in drug stores, health food stores and elsewhere is not diluted.

At least one physician, Dr. Hellfried Sartori of Rockville, Md., has been treating cancer patients with industrial strength DMSO. "To my knowledge, I'm the only successful cure for cancer," said Dr. Sartori, who charges $2,000 for 20-30 treatments, which are sometimes administered in his living room. Sartori is being investigated by the Maryland Commission on

Medical Discipline, which is concerned about his DMSO treatments and other unorthodox practices. "Because I'm different, they say I'm incompetent," Dr. Sartori said. "All I'm doing is helping patients." [20]

Dr. Stanley Jacob, associate professor of surgery at the University of Oregon and one of the leading DMSO advocates, has been charged in federal court with four counts of conspiracy and giving a gratuity in connection with charges that he paid $48,200 to an FDA official in charge of regulating DMSO. The FDA medical officer, Dr. K. C. Pani, is also under indictment for accepting money and falsifying DMSO study data. Drs. Jacob and Pani both have pleaded not guilty to the charges.

Preliminary Results of Interferon Research

One cancer treatment that has shown promise in recent years is immunotherapy, which uses substances produced naturally in the body to fight cancer. Immunotherapy backers admit, however, that it will be some time before this type of treatment is used successfully on a wide scale. "There is no form of immunotherapy that can be considered as established, conventional treatment," said Dr. Alexander Fefer, an immunologist and chief oncologist at the University of Washington in Seattle. "Every immunotherapy approach remains experimental." [21]

The type of immunotherapy that has received the most attention involves interferon, a protein that was first isolated in 1956. "Interferon is a sinuous, sticky protein," wrote Michael Edlehart, co-author of a book on the substance. "Virtually all human and animal cells are capable of manufacturing it, yet they do so only rarely and then in such minute quantities that detection takes enormous laboratory time.... The protein's existence has been known for 24 years, but it has been so hard to come by during that time that research has been difficult when not impossible." [22]

Preliminary tests begun in 1978 and sponsored by a $2 million grant from the American Cancer Society showed that 30 percent to 50 percent of cancer patients responded favorably to interferon treatment. This promising data, researchers cautioned, was preliminary and inconclusive. Much more extensive research is currently being carried out both in the United States and Europe. The American Cancer Society has allocated $4.3 million for interferon studies at 10 research institutes.

[20] Quoted in *The Washington Post*, Dec. 12, 1981.
[21] Quoted in *The New York Times*, April 14, 1981.
[22] Writing in *The New York Times Magazine*, April 26, 1981, p. 35. Edelhart's book, *Interferon: The New Hope for Cancer* (1981), was written with Dr. Jean Lindenmann, the Swiss researcher who first isolated interferon in 1956 while working at Britain's National Institute for Medical Research with British researcher Alcik Isaacs. Lindenmann and Isaacs published their discovery in 1957.

Interferon researchers are heartened by recent progress in genetic engineering. The hope is that biologists will be able to produce synthetically grown interferon in laboratories in large quantities so that extensive tests on cancer patients can be carried out. "Biologists have been able to splice the gene for human interferon production into the nuclear material of a bacterial cell," wrote Dr. Fitzhugh Mullan, a physician and scholar in residence at the Institute of Medicine. "The bacterium becomes a tiny factory for the production of the substance. The technology is new and far from being debugged, but its very existence makes interferon more like penicillin and less like a moon landing. Genetically produced interferon is currently undergoing its first human clinical trials, and it seems that within a few years it will be readily available in a pure and potent form." [23]

Monoclonal Antibodies and Hyperthermia

Another promising form of immunological cancer treatment that uses genetic engineering technology involves substances called monoclonal antibodies. They are made by fusing two different cells (a disease-fighting cell and a cancer cell), cloning them and then injecting them into the body to try to fight cancer. The first tests of monoclonal antibodies were carried out at the Stanford University Medical Center in California and by a group of researchers working at the Farber Cancer Institute and the Children's Hospital in Boston. "What we've all found is that monoclonal antibodies can cause a remarkable drop in cancer cells," said Dr. Stuart Schlossman of the Boston group.[24] But Schlossman and others caution that the technology is still very new. In spite of initial successes, a method has not been developed that always gets the antibodies to reach and eradicate cancer cells. Nor have scientists been able to create a monoclonal antibody that has kept its cancer-cell fighting abilities for long periods of time.

Experiments with heat therapy — hyperthermia — have been going on for decades. But only in recent years have doctors been able to use modern techniques to extend cancer patients' lives. Hyperthermia is based on the theory that cancer cells cannot withstand high temperatures because the cells impede circulation and heat stores up within them. Cancer specialists such as Dr. F. Kristian Storm at the University of California at Los Angeles have successfully treated some forms of cancer with heat. Dr. Storm uses heat-generating radio waves introduced to patients with a Magnetrode, a device that aims temperatures as

---

[23] Writing in *The Washington Post*, June 26, 1981. For background information see "Genetic Research," *E.R.R.*, 1977 Vol. I, pp. 223-244, and "Genetic Business," *E.R.R.*, 1980 Vol. II, pp. 945-964.
[24] Quoted in *The New York Times*, Aug. 31, 1981.

high as 122 degrees on cancerous tumors. In combination with chemotherapy, hyperthermia treatments with the Magnetrode have increased survival time for patients with skin cancer and cancer of the colon.

The Magnetrode accomplishes its work without bringing the sometimes unbearable heat to other, non-infected, parts of the body. "Hyperthermia is not a golden bullet [a term given to the hypothetical cancer treatment that will eradicate tumors without damaging another part of the body]," Dr. Storm said. "Alone it may help as a single agent for one-third of tumors that can be super-heated. Its greatest potential may be in combination with other therapies." [25]

Holistic Approach to Cancer Treatment

In recent years some cancer specialists have been adding other treatments to the traditional surgery, radiation and chemotherapy. These physicians practice holistic medicine. They treat the entire patient, not just the patient's cancer. The treatment can involve psychological counseling, biofeedback, nutrition counseling and other techniques. ". . . [I]llness is not purely a physical problem, but rather a problem of the whole person," said Dr. O. Carl Simonton, a radiation oncologist and director of the holistic Cancer Counseling and Research Center in Fort Worth, Texas. Simonton believes that illnesses such as cancer include "not only body but mind and emotions. We believe that emotional and mental states play a significant role both in *susceptibility* to disease, including cancer, and in *recovery* from all disease." [26]

In addition to receiving traditional therapies such as radiation, Simonton's patients are taught to envision their cancers and then to visualize their radiation treatments and their bodies' immunological systems fighting and defeating the cancer. Robin Casarjian, a Boston therapist who works with cancer patients using Simonton's and other holistic methods, described the holistic theory of treating cancer patients. "The theory assumes that everybody's body has cancer cells in it and the body also has its own mechanisms to deal with the cancer cells," she said in a recent interview. "It's a natural mechanism that functions within the immunological system. . . . To put it extremely simplistically: A psychological depression can cause a depression in the immune system. The opposite can also happen. As you gain a sense of control in your life, and see the power that you have and that the mind and body aren't separate, you can reverse what's happened in the body and the body can begin to heal itself."

---

[25] Quoted in *U.S. News & World Report,* April 6, 1981, p. 70.
[26] O. Carl Simonton, *et. al., Getting Well Again* (1978), p. 9.

The THC Connection

Nausea and vomiting are two of the unwanted side-effects of chemotherapy. Medical researchers do not know why chemotherapy causes these problems, but they have found a drug that is effective in relieving most cancer patients' chemically induced nausea and vomiting. The drug is delta-9-tetrahydrocannabinal (THC), the active ingredient in marijuana.

THC's effectiveness in relieving nausea and vomiting was first brought to the attention of cancer specialists in the mid-1970s by young patients who smoked marijuana. These early reports of marijuana's soothing effect brought about the first scientific experiments with THC and chemotherapy at the Sidney Farber Cancer Institute in Boston in 1975. The initial tests found that of the 22 young cancer patients receiving chemotherapy, 14 reported a significant lessening of nausea and vomiting after smoking marijuana. Three subsequent studies — at the Mayo Clinic, the National Cancer Institute (NCI) and the Farber Institute — confirmed the initial findings.

The Food and Drug Administration began allowing cancer patients to ingest THC capsules in September 1980. The capsules are ordered by oncologists (cancer specialists) through NCI-registered hospital pharmacies for patients who cannot use any other anti-nausea drugs. The reason for the special arrangements is that THC is classified as a "Schedule I controlled substance," an illegal drug.

The first cancer patient to smoke marijuana legally in New York did so on Dec. 16, 1981, at North Shore Hospital in Manhasset. "This is the first time I have not felt sick within two hours after my [chemo]therapy," the patient, Bonnie Adlman, told the New York *Daily News*. "Usually I'm sick as a dog by now."

Psychological counseling for patients and family members has become a part of cancer treatment at some of the nation's large cancer institutes. At Memorial Sloan-Kettering in New York, Dr. Jimmie Holland, chief of the psychiatric service, treats cancer patients for what she calls the five Ds: death, disfigurement, disability, dependence and disruption of relationships. "How a person deals with them is really what coping with cancer is all about," Dr. Holland said.[27]

Despite the recent advances in treating cancer patients and their families, the fact remains that of those persons diagnosed with cancer in 1982, only about half will live longer than five years. The immediate future promises more gains in treatment techniques. But cancer researchers still cannot foresee the day when they will discover the "magic bullet" that will cure most cancers.

---

[27] Quoted in *Newsweek*, Nov. 2, 1981, p. 98.

119

Selected Bibliography

Books

Brody, Jane and Arthur Holleb, *You Can Fight Cancer and Win,* Times Books, 1977.

Edelhart, Michael and Jean Lindenmann, *Interferon: The New Hope for Cancer,* Addison-Wesley, 1981.

McGrady, Pat, *The Savage Cell,* Basic Books, 1964.

Moss, Ralph W., *The Cancer Syndrome,* Grove Press, 1980.

Prescott, David M. and Abraham S. Flexer, *Cancer: The Misguided Cell,* Scribner's, 1982.

Richards, Victor, *Cancer, the Wayward Cell: Its Origins, Nature and Treatment,* University of California Press, 1972.

Sontag, Susan, *Illness as Metaphor,* Farrar, Straus and Giroux, 1977.

Whelan, Elizabeth M., *Preventing Cancer,* Norton, 1978.

Articles

Clark, Matt, *et al.,* "Cancer — A Progress Report," *Newsweek,* Nov. 2, 1981.

Journal of the National Cancer Institute, selected issues.

"Rooting Out Cancer," *The Economist,* Sept. 19, 1981.

Schepartz, Saul A., *et al.,* "New Approaches in Cancer Chemotherapy," *Pharmacy Times,* November 1981.

Science, selected issues.

Silk, Andrew, "The Struggle of Andrew Silk: A Young Man Confronts Cancer," *The New York Times Magazine,* Oct. 18, 1981.

Smart, Charles R., "Progress in Cancer Patient Management in Community Hospitals," *Bulletin of the American College of Surgeons,* September 1981.

Trafford, Abigail, "Latest Strides in Fight Against Cancer," *U.S. News & World Report,* April 6, 1981.

Reports and Studies

American Cancer Society, "Cancer Facts and Figures, 1982," 1981.

American Council on Science and Health, "Cancer in the United States: Is There an Epidemic?" August 1980.

Editorial Research Reports: "Strategies for Controlling Cancer," 1977 Vol. II, p. 577; "Quest for Cancer Control," 1974 Vol. II, p. 623; "Cancer Research Progress," 1967 Vol. I, p. 221.

Leukemia Society of America, "Annual Report, 1981," 1981.

National Cancer Institute, "Surveillance, Epidemiology and End Results: Incidence and Mortality Data, 1973-77," June 1981.

National Institutes of Health, "Decade of Discovery: Advances in Cancer Research," October 1981; "Chemotherapy and You: A Guide to Self-Help During Treatment," November 1980.

Cover illustration by Staff Artist Robert Redding

CONTROVERSY OVER SALT IN FOOD

by

Marc Leepson

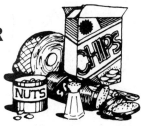

**Dec. 11
1 9 8 1**

Editor's Note: The bill introduced by Reps. Gore and Smith to require processed food containing more than 35 milligrams of sodium per average serving to show the amount on the label *(p. 134)* never was enacted by Congress. The Food and Drug Administration continues to encourage the food industry to label sodium content voluntarily and about one-third of the processed foods the agency regulates is now labeled for sodium, according to a report released by the FDA July 15, 1983. Thus far, the effort by the Reagan administration to overhaul the nation's food safety laws and do away with the Delaney Clause *(p. 138)* has not succeeded, although congressional hearings have been held on the issue. Congress voted last May to extend the prohibition on banning the artificial sweetener saccharin until June 30, 1985 *(see p. 139)*.

CONTROVERSY OVER SALT IN FOOD

SALT is a big issue in Washington these days. That's salt with a small "s," the kind you sprinkle on food. Salt is the second leading food additive (behind sugar), and Americans consume a lot of it, an average of two to five teaspoons per day. It is the sodium content of salt that concerns health officials.[1] Faced with mounting evidence linking excessive sodium consumption to hypertension (high blood pressure), the government has begun a campaign to get Americans to reduce their salt intake.

"During roughly the last 10 years there has been a gradual development of what I would call a national medical and biological consensus about the association between sodium and blood pressure," said Dr. Allan L. Forbes, associate director for nutrition and food sciences in the Food and Drug Administration's Bureau of Foods. "That consensus has become national only in the last year or two."[2]

About 60 million Americans suffer from some form of hypertension. This includes a high percentage of blacks, about 37 percent, and those over 65, about 40 percent. Those who do not keep their blood pressure under control face an increased risk of strokes, heart attacks and kidney problems. High blood pressure is the primary cause of the approximately half-million cases of stroke and 170,000 stroke deaths that occur annually. And hypertension is a factor in many of the 1.25 million heart attacks suffered by Americans each year and the 650,000 heart attack deaths.

Medical researchers are quick to point out that there is no conclusive proof that sodium causes hypertension. Nevertheless, the medical evidence to date indicates what appears to be a strong relationship between sodium consumption and high blood pressure, and physicians routinely put hypertensive patients and recuperating heart attack victims on low-sodium or sodium-free diets. "Right now we don't know precisely what role sodium plays in people with high blood pressure or why some people are more sensitive to salt than others," Richard S. Schweiker, secretary of health and human services, told rep-

---

[1] Table salt is composed of 40 percent sodium and 60 percent chlorine (see p. 128).
[2] Quoted in *FDA Consumer*, October 1981, p. 11.

resentatives of the food processing industry at a June 30, 1981, meeting in Washington, D.C., sponsored by the Food and Drug Administration (FDA). "We do know, however, that while sodium does not necessarily cause high blood pressure, it does aggravate it. . . . For people with high blood pressure or the disposition to get it, [sodium] can be unhealthy."

FDA Commissioner Arthur Hull Hayes Jr. is one of the leading advocates of reduced sodium consumption. Hayes, a physician who took over as head of the agency on April 13, 1981, was director of the Hypertension Clinic at the Hershey (Pa.) Medical Center. "We know that it is easier to treat many patients with hypertension if their salt intake is reduced," Hayes said at the June 30 meeting. "We know that many people with mild hypertension show a significant fall . . . in terms of risk if they reduce their sodium. This is not to say that we understand everything about sodium and the genesis of hypertension. But if we wait until we understand everything about a disease before we start attacking those problems . . . then obviously a lot of people are going to remain sick that needn't."

Medical Findings Spur Public Response

The first medical evidence linking sodium and hypertension was uncovered 77 years ago.[3] Since then, dozens of studies throughout the world have found that societies that consume very small amounts of sodium — such as the primitive peoples of the Amazon Basin, New Guinea, rural Uganda and Alaska — have exceedingly low rates of hypertension. Conversely, those societies that ingest large amounts of sodium — such as the northern Japanese who consume an average of 13 teaspoons of salt daily — have the highest hypertension rates in the world.

The U.S. Senate Select Committee on Nutrition and Human Needs, in a February 1977 report on "Dietary Goals for the United States," was the first federal body to recommend that Americans reduce salt consumption. Two years later the U.S. surgeon general and a Task Force on Hypertension Research at the National Heart, Lung and Blood Institute recommended a reduction in salt intake as a way to help prevent disease. The National Academy of Science's Food and Nutrition Board joined the chorus in its May 1980 report "Toward Healthful Diets." The American Medical Association and the American Heart Association also have recommended that Americans reduce sodium consumption.

Several years ago the Food and Drug Administration commissioned a special committee of the Federation of the American Societies for Experimental Biology (FASEB) to evaluate the

---

[3] In 1904, two French medical researchers, L. Ambard and and E. Beaujard, published the first data linking salt and hypertension in a French medical journal.

health implications of salt as a food additive. The FASEB report, issued in 1979, concluded: "It is the prevalent judgment of the scientific community that the consumption of sodium chloride in the aggregate should be lowered in the United States." The report recommended that FDA establish guidelines for restricting the amount of salt in processed foods. According to Dr. Mark Novitch, acting FDA deputy commissioner, the findings of the FASEB report raise "questions about the safety of sodium chloride at current levels of use."[4]

The American public apparently has taken note of these warnings. In a poll commissioned last year by the Chicago advertising agency Foote, Cone and Belding, 42 percent of those surveyed said they were avoiding the use of salt in foods.[5] A more extensive survey was conducted by the U.S. Department of Agriculture's Economics and Statistics Service between November 1979 and January 1980 to find out how consumers' views on health and nutrition affected their food consumption. Five percent of the 1,353 households surveyed said they never used salty foods or snacks, and 21 percent said they were cutting down on salty foods.

Nearly 30 percent of those who reported making diet changes for health or nutritional reasons said they were concerned about reducing salt intake or controlling blood pressure. A large majority of those surveyed (86 percent) agreed that increased salt consumption heightened the risk of high blood pressure. Those concerned about salt consumption, the survey found, also used less white bread, diet soft drinks, artificial sweeteners and snacks such as potato chips, corn chips and pretzels. Those same persons used more poultry, fish, lowfat milk, corn oil margarine and whole-grain bread.[6]

Debate Over Minimum Requirements

The human body needs sodium to maintain blood pressure and volume and to control water passage through the body. Excessive salt loss through perspiration in extremely hot weather can lead to heat exhaustion, cramps and, in extreme cases, death from heat prostration, especially in children and the elderly. The minimal amount of sodium needed to maintain health varies from person to person, depending upon body weight.

Medical experts say that the daily minimum is 200-400 milli-

---

[4] Testifying before the Subcommittee on Investigations and Oversight of the House Science and Technology Committee, April 14, 1981.
[5] The survey was taken in March 1980. Of 700 persons surveyed, 292 answered "yes" to the question, "In the food you eat, do you cut down on salt and sodium?"
[6] See Judy Jones and Jon Weimer, "Perspective on Health Related Food Choices," U.S. Department of Agriculture, National Economics Division, Economics and Statistics Service, Nov. 19, 1980.

grams — an amount most persons get from sodium found naturally in food and water. "What is frightening is how little sodium our body needs," said FDA Commissioner Hayes. "In fact, the only sodium we need is the amount we lose every day. And that is really a rather small amount."

The Salt Institute, the industry's trade association, contends that an average daily sodium intake of 4,000 to 4,800 milligrams "is not harmful to healthy individuals. The healthy body adjusts to varying salt intake by excreting the excess salt and has the ability to retain only the amount of sodium it needs."[7] The Food and Nutrition Board of the National Academy of Sciences reports that daily sodium intakes of 1,100 to 3,300 milligrams are "safe and adequate" for the healthy adult. But the typical American consumes 10 to 20 times that amount. One reason Americans' sodium intake is so high is that a number of widely used chemically manufactured food additives contain sodium.

'Hidden' Sources of Sodium in the Diet

Salt applied to food at the table makes up only about a third of all sodium consumed. Nearly half of Americans' sodium intake comes from "hidden" sources — processed foods such as canned and dried soups, canned vegetables, pickles, olives, canned tuna and crab, sauerkraut and frozen dinners. Large quantities of sodium also are found in foods that are not "salty," such as instant puddings, cereals, ice cream, cookies, cakes and breads *(see chart, p. 130)*. Since food processors are not required to list sodium content on their labels *(see p. 134)*, it is often difficult for those on low-sodium diet sto know if the foods they eat contain large amounts of sodium.

Different brands of the same foods can have significantly different amounts of sodium. According to information compiled by nutritionist Bonnie Liebman of the Center for Science in the Public Interest, some of the best-selling brands of breads, processed meats, frozen foods, canned vegetables and fast foods contain much more sodium than other brands. One brand of tomato paste, for example, has no added salt, while another uses 700 milligrams in a six-ounce can. One brand of English muffin contains 633 milligrams of sodium, another 290. Most food processing companies "use as much salt as their recipes call for," Liebman said, "without a second thought about trying to minimize those levels."[8]

Food processors say that the amount of salt added to pro-

---

[7] See the Salt Institute's pamphlet, "Salt Tidbits: Some Answers on Salt," 1979.
[8] Quoted in *National Journal*, Oct. 17, 1981, p. 1865. Also see "How Salt Creeps Into Daily Diets," *Nutrition Action*, April 1981.

cessed foods reflects consumer taste. "The seasoning of foods with salt is, of course, a historical and traditional practice, both in the home and in the processing plant to the extent necessary to achieve consumer acceptance," said Fritz C. Friday, president of a Wisconsin canning corporation and a former chairman of the National Food Processors Association. "Not all consumers, of course, like exactly the same amount of salt in a given food, and accordingly not all commercial brands are designed to contain the same salt concentration. Regional, ethnic and other factors may also dictate variations in the addition of salt to processed foods."[9]

Dr. Henry Blackburn, chairman of the Department of Physiological Hygiene at the University of Minnesota, contends that the nation's salty tooth has been nurtured by eating patterns begun in childhood. "Our salt appetite is culturally determined, not physiologically regulated," Blackburn said at a Feb. 25, 1981, news conference in Washington sponsored by the Center for Science in the Public Interest. "These high levels of sodium intake are created and maintained by the introduction of salt to infant foods, by the heavy salting used in food processing, by the highly salted snack foods, and by food traditions."

There are several ways to shake the salt habit. The best methods, nutritionists say, are to avoid eating processed foods or to choose those that contain low amounts of sodium. A cup of fresh lima beans, for example, contains only 2 milligrams of sodium; a cup of canned limas has 456 milligrams. A half pound of raw potatoes has about 5 milligrams of sodium; a half pound of frozen French fries has about 500. Most grocery and health-food stores offer low-sodium or sodium-free prepared foods. These products, known as special dietary foods, must have their sodium content listed on their labels.

Salt substitutes are sold in grocery stores, but some dietary experts warn that these substances contain high amounts of potassium and other additives that may be dangerous to those who should avoid sodium. Selling additive-laden salt substitutes "is something like selling 'lite' beer and 'lite' whiskey to alcoholics," food writers John and Karen Hess contend. One salt substitute, they said, "is half salt and half potassium chloride, calcium polysilicate, magnesium carbonate, and dextrose (sugar). It tastes fairly bitter and medicinal, which may be a selling point."[10] A number of cookbooks, including the American Heart Association's *Cooking Without Your Salt Shaker* (1978), provide instructions for low-sodium and sodium-free

[9] Testifying before the Subcommittee on Health and the Environment of the House Committee on Energy and Commerce, Sept. 25, 1981.
[10] John L. Hess and Karen Hess, *The Taste of America* (1977), p. 281.

cooking. These books suggest using spices, herbs, lemon or lime juice as food flavorings rather than salt. Craig Claiborne, food editor of *The New York Times,* told a congressional subcommittee that there are many ways that "one can substitute foods, spices and flavoring that will compensate for the lack of salt" in the diet.[11]

History and Usage of Salt

HISTORIANS believe that man was using salt as a food preservative and seasoning before recorded history. The earliest published reference to salt is found in a Chinese treatise on pharmacology written around 2,700 B.C. Salt was an extremely valued commodity in Greek and Roman times. Both civilizations offered salt to their gods and used salt as a food preservative. The Romans also used salt as payment for soldiers, a system called *salarium argentum,* from which the word "salary" is derived. There are more than 20 references to salt in the Bible, including the often-quoted phrase "salt of the earth" (Matthew V, 13).

Throughout history the use of salt has been associated with agricultural peoples rather than nomadic tribes. Most American Indians, for example, were hunters and avoided using salt. More domesticated Indian tribes in the southwest traveled to the Great Salt Lake in what is now Utah to gather salt for use as a trading commodity and as a flavoring for corn, squash and beans.

Salt was an important commodity in the American colonies. Sea-salt processing plants were established from Massachusetts to New Jersey during the Revolutionary War after the British shut off supplies from abroad. A noted British accomplishment during the war came in October 1777 when Gen. William Howe captured George Washington's salt supply in Philadelphia. Salt has figured in other political events, including the French Revolution, which was caused in part by the French people's revolt against increased salt taxes.

There are many different kinds of salts, all of which are chemical compounds. Common table salt, the compound sodium chloride (NaCl), is composed of 40 percent sodium and 60 percent chlorine. In their elemental states sodium and chlorine

---

[11] Testifying April 13, 1981, before the House Science and Technology Subcommittee on Investigations and Oversight.
[12] See the Salt Institute's "Facts About Salt: History, Production, Uses," 1980.

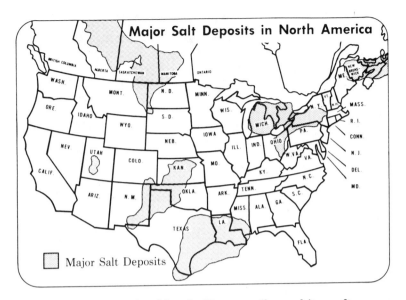

Major Salt Deposits in North America

☐ Major Salt Deposits

are extremely unpalatable. Sodium, a silver-white soft waxy element of the alkali metal group, is very active chemically. It combines with many other chemicals to form a number of products, including sodium bicarbonate (baking soda) and sodium fluoride (the agent used in water fluoridation). Chlorine, a toxic greenish yellow gas, has a very strong odor and is used most commonly as a bleach, oxidizing agent and disinfectant in water purification.

Production Methods and Industry Uses

All salt originated as sea salt. The ancient sea beds that covered the world 300 million years ago evaporated eons ago, but they left vast underground deposits of salt in many areas. Salt today is produced by underground mining, by evaporating sea water or by solution mining — pumping water into a salt deposit and then bringing it to the surface where it is evaporated in large vacuum pans.

Salt mining is similar to coal mining. A shaft is sunk into the ground to reach the salt beds, which are located from 600 to 2,000 feet below the surface. Miners hammer out salt from the mine walls, and the salt is carried to the surface where the rock salt is crushed and reduced. Some salt beds are circular, dome-shaped structures. The world's tallest salt domes are found below the surface of Louisiana and Texas. Some descend 55,000 feet into the earth and are more than a mile wide.

Most salt domes contain 99 percent sodium chloride. Large salt beds are found beneath thousands of square miles of Michigan, New York, Ohio, Pennsylvania, Kansas, Oklahoma, Texas and Louisiana *(see map, above)*. Other areas with large salt

129

What You Might Not See on the Label...

	Portion	Weight (grams)	Sodium (in milligrams)
Dairy Products			
Cheddar cheese	1 oz.	28	176
Cottage cheese	4 oz.	113	457
Swiss cheese	1 oz.	28	213
American cheese	1 oz.	28	406
Milk, whole or fat	1 cup	244	122
Yogurt, plain, lowfat	8 oz.	227	159
Egg	1 egg	50	59
Fish and Shellfish			
Herring, smoked	3 oz.	85	5,234
Sardines, canned	3 oz.	85	552
Tuna, canned (light meat, chunk, water pack)	3 oz.	85	288
Shrimp, canned	3 oz.	85	1,955
Meat and Poultry			
Corned beef	3 oz.	85	802
Bacon	2 slices	14	274
Chicken, breast with skin, roasted	½ breast	98	69
Chicken, canned	5 oz. can	142	714
Frankfurter	1	57	639
Chili con carne with beans, canned	1 cup	255	1,194
Frozen beef dinner	1 dinner	312	998
Beef pot pie	1 pie	227	1,093
Canned spaghetti and meatballs	7.5 oz.	213	942
Fast food cheeseburger	1 each	111	709
Fast food chicken dinner	1 portion	410	2,243
Fruit			
Cherries, raw	1 cup	150	1
Cherries, canned	1 cup	257	10
Peaches, raw	1 peach	100	1
Peaches, canned	1 cup	256	15
Pineapple, raw	1 cup	135	1
Pineapple, canned	1 cup	255	7
Pasta, Bread, Grains			
White bread	1 slice	25	114
Rye bread	1 slice	25	139
Cheerios	1¼ cup	28	304
Granola	¼ cup	34	61
Wheaties	1 cup	28	355

... Sodium Content of Selected Foods

	Portion	Weight (grams)	Sodium (in milligrams)
Pancake mix	1 cup	141	2,036
Stuffing mix, cooked	1 cup	170	1,131
Vegetables			
Lima beans, cooked	1 cup	170	2
Lima beans, canned	1 cup	170	456
Corn, cooked	1 ear	140	1
Corn, canned	1 cup	165	384
Mushrooms, raw	1 cup	70	7
Mushrooms, canned	2 oz.	56	242
Peas, cooked	1 cup	160	2
Peas, frozen	3 oz.	85	80
Tomatoes, raw	1 tomato	123	14
Tomatoes, canned whole	1 cup	240	390
Tomato sauce	1 cup	248	1,498
Condiments			
Baking powder	1 tsp.	3	339
Baking soda	1 tsp.	3	821
Catsup	1 tbsp.	15	156
Garlic salt	1 tsp.	6	1,850
MSG (monosodium glutamate)	1 tsp.	5	1,750
Mustard, prepared	1 tsp.	5	65
Olives, green	4 olives	16	323
Onion salt	1 tsp.	5	1,620
Pickles, dill	1 pickle	65	928
Salt	1 tsp.	5	1,938
A-1 sauce	1 tbsp.	17	275
Soy sauce	1 tbsp.	18	1,029
Tabasco sauce	1 tsp.	5	24
Worcestershire	1 tbsp.	17	206
Legumes and nuts			
Almonds, salted, roasted	1 cup	157	311
Boston style baked beans	1 cup	260	606
Kidney beans, dry cooked	1 cup	182	4
Kidney beans, canned	1 cup	255	844
Cashews, dry roasted, salted	1 cup	140	1,200
Peanuts, dry roasted, salted	1 cup	144	986
Peanuts, roasted, salted	1 cup	144	601
Peanuts, Spanish, salted	1 cup	144	823
Peanuts, unsalted	1 cup	144	8
Peanut butter	1 tbsp.	16	81

Source: U.S. Department of Agriculture

deposits are found in the British Isles, the Soviet Union, China, India, France, West Germany, Italy and Canada.

Solution mining uses what is known as a brine well. An underground salt deposit is flooded with water and the brine (salty water) is piped to the surface where it undergoes heat processing. Natural brines exist throughout the world. The largest in this country are in Michigan, New York, Ohio, Pennsylvania and Utah's Great Salt Lake. Others are in Austria, France, Germany, India and the enormous Dead Sea on the boundary between Israel and Jordan.

According to the Salt Institute, the United States produces about 26 million tons of dry salt and 23 million tons of brine a year. Salt is used in more than 14,000 different ways, but only 5 percent of the salt mined in this country is used in food processing. The chemical industry — especially the glass, soap, glaze and enamel segments — uses about 70 percent of the U.S. supply. Salt is used to produce hundreds of different chemical products, including paper, detergents, plastics, synthetic rubber and synthetic fabrics.

The Salt Institute estimates that about 13.1 million tons of salt are poured on roads and highways every year in North America to break down snow and ice. Some three million tons of salt are used annually in water softening, primarily in the textile, leather and laundry industries. Nearly 2 million tons are used each year in U.S. agriculture, primarily as a food additive in animal feed. Salt also is widely used as a road building material since it helps stabilize soil on road beds, rural roads and highway shoulders.

Extra Ingredients in Common Table Salt

Salt is used in many different ways by the food industry — as a flavor and processing ingredient in hundreds of canned and frozen foods, a curing agent in meat and fish, a leavener in bread and as an inhibiter of bacteria growth in bacon, sausage and bread. What is known as "table salt" is made up of fine crystals that have been baked at 1,200 degrees Fahrenheit and then quickly cooled.

Although table salt is 99.99 percent sodium chloride, it contains some additives. Since 1924 potassium iodide has been added to salt to prevent endemic goiter, a swelling of the thyroid gland caused by insufficient iodine in the diet. Not all table salts contain iodine; those that do are marked on the label. Since the introduction of iodine, goiter has been nearly eliminated in this country.

Iodine is only one of the additives found in table salt. Because iodine oxidizes rapidly when exposed to light, salt manufacturers add a stabilizer, usually dextrose, a simple sugar. The Salt Institute estimates that dextrose makes up 0.0374 percent of table salt. Sodium silico aluminate is often added to keep table salt freely flowing. Sodium bicarbonate is used to bleach out the purple color of the potassium iodide. Some salts contain calcium carbonate, a naturally occurring compound that prevents caking.

Controlling Sodium Intake

NEARLY EVERYONE agrees that Americans consume too much salt and that sodium intake should be reduced. There are disagreements, however, over how best to help Americans reduce their salt consumption. On Feb. 25, 1981, more than 5,000 health professionals and students organized by the Center for Science in the Public Interest submitted a petition to the Food and Drug Administration asking the agency to limit sodium in processed foods. "The problem is less a scientific than a practical dilemma," said Dr. Henry Blackburn of the University of Minnesota, one of the petition's signatories. "The problem is how can the individual avoid excess sodium when so much is added to food before it reaches the table?"[13]

The Food and Drug Administration had been under pressure for several years from consumer groups to limit sodium in processed foods and to have the sodium content of foods shown on labels. But not until Arthur Hayes Jr. became FDA commissioner did the agency move on the issue. Hayes, a physician who specialized in treating hypetension *(see p. 124)*, has strong views on the subject. "It is rather frustrating for a physician to advise patients with hypertension to avoid foods that contain large amounts of sodium, and then have the patient go out and eat foods without knowing how much sodium they actually contain," Hayes told representatives of the food processing industry at a June 30 meeting in Washington. "Many of my patients expressed interest in having sodium content labeling on foods, as well as a greater variety and number of processed foods from which to choose, and I'm delighted to be in a position to do something about it."

What Hayes did was apply the Reagan administration's anti-regulatory philosophy to the issue. Instead of advocating mandatory government action, Hayes asked the food processing industry to reduce the sodium in processed foods voluntarily, to

---

[13] Quoted in *Nutrition Action*, April 1981, p. 3.

market a wider variety of low-sodium products and to work with the government to develop consumer information programs about the dangers of consuming too much sodium. The agency also asked the industry to list sodium content on the nutrition labels of processed foods and to help work out definitions of the terms "low sodium" and "moderately low sodium."

FDA representatives have met with industry groups to explore ways to help the public understand the relationship between sodium and hypertension. The agency also is monitoring U.S. sodium consumption. Hayes told the House Subcommittee on Health and the Environment Sept. 25 that the voluntary effort will "dramatically increase the amount of sodium information [available to consumers] over the next several years." Hayes said he would support legislation ordering mandatory sodium labeling "only if voluntary efforts on the part of the food industry fail."

Voluntary vs. Mandatory Sodium Labeling

Hayes was testifying at a hearing on a bill introduced by Reps. Albert Gore Jr., D-Tenn., and Neal Smith, D-Iowa, that would require processed food containing more than 35 milligrams of sodium per average serving to show the amount on the label. "I do not claim that sodium labeling alone will 'cure' high blood pressure," Rep. Gore said at the Sept. 25 hearing, "but I do believe that it can play a useful role in controlling the very bad health outcomes from the disease."

On the question of voluntary labeling, Gore said: "I believe that the facts in the sodium case argue strongly that voluntarism alone will not work to provide the American people with the information they need. . . . In the case of sodium labeling, where various companies perceive distinct competitive disadvantages to disclosure, it is reasonable to expect much slower implementation of important public health information if it is left to voluntary implementation. I would not be surprised to see voluntary sodium labeling take 15 years before it grabbed hold in the market."

Representatives of the Center for Science in the Public Interest, the American Heart Association and the American Medical Association also testified in support of mandatory sodium content labeling. Philip L. White, director of the AMA's department of foods and nutrition, said his association would support a voluntary industry-wide program, but in the absence of such a plan, the AMA favors a mandatory approach. "Without information regarding sodium content labeling, dietary planning by physicians and their patients is more difficult," White said. "Obviously, a cost-effective system of sodium labeling for foods

Sodium in Water and Drugs

Tap water, unless it has been distilled or demineralized, contains sodium. The amount varies depending on geographical region. Tap water in Newark, N.J., for example, contains 10 milligrams of sodium per eight ounces; in Miami Beach, it is 13 milligrams; in Dallas, 14; and in San Diego, 15.

Non-distilled bottled waters — mineral waters, club sodas and seltzers — also contain varying amounts of sodium. Some bottled waters have less sodium than some public water systems. Perrier, imported from France, has only two milligrams of sodium per eight ounces compared to some club sodas that have as much as 60 milligrams.

Some over-the-counter drugs contain large amounts of sodium. Among the higher concentrations in popular non-prescription drugs are:

Drug	Milligrams per dose
Bromo-Seltzer	717
Alka-Seltzer (blue box)	521
Alka-Seltzer Antacid (gold box)	276
Sal Hepatica (laxative)	1,000
Brioschi (antacid)	710
Miles Nervine Effervescent (sleep aid)	544

would be beneficial to both physicians and their patients and would thus be of considerable assistance in the dietary management of hypertension."

Salt Institute President William E. Dickinson told the subcommittee that his organization was against mandatory labeling primarily because such a law would put financial strains on some food processors. Soft-drink manufacturers, for example, would have a difficult and costly time calculating their products' sodium content because the amount of sodium in water varies depending on geographical location. Fritz C. Friday, former chairman of the National Food Processors Association, said food companies would have to buy additional equipment to measure sodium content, revise their labels, maintain a large label supply and recall products ruled unacceptable. Paul F. Hopper, corporate director of scientific affairs for General Foods Corp., which has begun sodium labeling on some of its products, told the subcommittee that small businesses lack the "laboratory facilities ... to assure compliance with label declaration, batch after batch, week after week."

Recent Evidence of Industry Cooperation

FDA Commissioner Hayes said last September[14] that he would know "within six to 10 months" whether the voluntary

[14] Testifying Sept. 25, 1981, before the House Subcommittee on Health and the Environment.

program was working. Less than two months later, Hayes told a meeting of the National Health Council in Washington that the voluntary effort "has had a measure of success." Hayes said at the Nov. 11 meeting that "a number of companies have indicated they will label their foods with sodium information and explore low-sodium foods. . . ." FDA's Bureau of Foods estimates that by next spring as many as 40 percent of the processed foods on the market will have some form of sodium labeling. "This is a threefold increase from the amount of sodium labeling among processed foods when our voluntary effort began," Hayes said, calling the situation a "demonstration of support and response from the food industry."

"It is rather frustrating for a physician to advise patients with hypertension to avoid foods that contain large amounts of sodium, and then have the patient go out and eat foods without knowing how much sodium they actually contain."

Dr. Arthur Hayes Jr., FDA
Commissioner, June 30, 1981

The Food and Drug Administration held meetings with food industry representatives, food companies and trade associations throughout 1981. As a result of those meetings, the American Meat Institute, the National Soft Drink Association, the National Food Processors Association, the American Frozen Food Institute and other groups pledged to work with their members on sodium labeling. A number of food processors already offer products with the sodium content labeled. And some, including the Campbell Soup Co., are marketing reduced sodium and sodium-free products. Campbell began reducing sodium in its soups after marketing surveys indicated that more than half the population was concerned about sodium in food. The Jewel Food Stores, a Chicago-based supermarket chain, introduced four private-label "no salt added" fruit and vegetable items last April.

Giant Food, a 128-supermarket chain in the Baltimore-Washington area, has begun listing the sodium content on the labels of some of its house brands. In addition, the chain's "in-store" consumer awareness program includes free pamphlets on the dangers of excess sodium consumption. Oscar Meyer, a recent acquisition of General Foods Corp., has begun listing sodium content on the nutrition statements on some of its products;

Types of Salt

Evaporated Salt is produced by open pan or vacuum pan evaporation of brine under conditions designed to control crystal size and purity.

Solar Salt is produced by evaporation of sea, salt lake or underground saline waters by sun and wind in shallow ponds.

Rock Salt. A mineral halite (sodium chloride) occurring in the form of rock masses and beds.

Table Salt. Evaporated salt produced for human consumption, available plain or iodized.

Iodized Salt has a minute amount of potassium iodide added to prevent goiter.

Trace Mineralized Salt. Salt in either loose, brick or 50-pound block form that has minute amounts of trace minerals added; used in livestock feeding.

Water Softener Salt. High quality, either rock, solar or compressed, evaporated in pellet or block form, used to regenerate water softening systems.

Sea Salt is produced from sea water, same as solar salt.

Popcorn Salt. Fine particles of evaporated salt, used in seasoning popcorn.

Pretzel Salt. A coarse salt used in making pretzels.

Ice Cream Salt. Usually rock salt, used to enhance the freezing process in making ice cream.

Deicing Salt, either in rock or solar form, is used to melt ice and snow on roads in winter.

Canning Salt. Plain evaporated salt with no additives.

Pickling Salt. Same as canning salt.

Flour Salt. A super-fine grade of salt for use in cake mixes and other commercial baking.

Kosher Salt. A coarse evaporated salt produced for use in Kosher foods.

Enriched Bakers' Salt contains thiamine, riboflavin, niacin and iron and is used in commercial baking.

Source: Salt Institute

items with less-than 35 milligrams of sodium per serving are not labeled. An informal survey of supermarket shelves by the Salt Institute found that most cereal manufacturers had begun labeling sodium content in milligrams per serving and milligrams per 100 grams.

Congressional Review of Food Safety Laws

The Food and Drug Administration is not the only government agency trying to get the food industry to reduce voluntarily the amount of sodium in processed foods. The U.S. Department of Agriculture (USDA), which regulates meat and dairy products, has been cooperating closely with the FDA to encourage the meat and poultry processing industries to reduce sodium amounts and to begin using labels listing sodium content. The department's Food Safety and Inspection Service has begun what it calls an "urgent" program to study how to lower the sodium in some meat and poultry products by at least 25 percent. Researchers will examine luncheon meats, bacon and ham, as well as chicken and turkey frankfurters, which are 35-45 percent higher in sodium than beef franks. According to USDA calculations, the sodium content of cooked ham has risen as much as 40 percent since 1965.[15]

"In the case of sodium labeling, where various companies perceive distinct competitive disadvantages to disclosure, it is reasonable to expect much slower implementation of important public health information if it is left to voluntary implementation."

Rep. Albert Gore Jr., D-Tenn.
Sept. 25, 1981

The government's interest in sodium content comes at a time when the nation's food safety laws are being challenged by the food industry and its supporters in Congress and the Reagan administration. A bill pending in Congress that is thought to have a good chance of passing next year would substantially change the way the government handles food safety. Its primary target is the so-called Delaney Clause, which prohibits the use of any food additive found to induce cancer in animals or humans even if some putatively safe level for human food could be established. Use of such additives is thus prohibited.[16] Industry officials say this absolute prohibition is unrealistic. Instead, they want federal regulators to concentrate on those substances that pose a "significant risk" to health.

Interest in rewriting the food safety laws grew principally out of controversies in recent years over two substances that laboratory tests had linked to cancer: the artificial sweetener saccharin and the meat preservative sodium nitrite. The FDA tried to ban saccharin in 1977 after laboratory tests conducted in Canada showed that some rats developed bladder cancer after being fed a heavy diet of the substance. Soon after the proposed ban was announced, Congress was deluged by protests from diabetics, dieters, the soft-drink industry and other saccharin supporters. Congress responded by prohibiting any ban on saccharin pend-

---

[15] See *Food Engineering,* October 1981, pp. 31-32.
[16] See "Food Additives," *E.R.R.,* 1978 Vol. I, pp. 341-360, and *Congressional Quarterly Weekly Report,* Sept. 19, 1981, pp. 1791-1793.

ing further studies, but requiring warning labels on products containing the substance. The congressional prohibition has been extended several times, most recently last summer when Congress approved legislation continuing it until June 30, 1983.

After a study suggested that sodium nitrite caused cancer in laboratory animals, the FDA in 1978 began action against the preservative. The agency sought to phase out rather than ban the use of nitrite because there was no ready substitute to guard against botulism, the deadly food poisoning. The Carter administration asked Congress in April 1979 for special legislation delaying any regulatory action for at least a year, but Congress did not take action on that request. Finally, in August 1980, government officials withdrew their actions against sodium nitrite, saying that subsequent laboratory testing did not confirm that the substance was carcinogenic.

In the case of sodium, nearly all medical experts agree that excessive consumption presents a significant health risk. Whether or not food safety laws are rewritten, the government is likely to continue to encourage people to cut down on sodium consumption.

Selected Bibliography

Books

Cooking Without Your Salt Shaker, American Heart Association, 1978.

Health Policy: The Legislative Agenda, Congressional Quarterly, 1980.

Hess, John and Karen Hess, *The Taste of America*, Penguin Books, 1977.

Hinich, Melvin J. and Richard Staelin, *Consumer Protection Legislation and the U.S. Food Industry*, Pergamon Press, 1980.

Kaufman, Dale W., ed., *Sodium Chloride*, Rheinholt, 1960.

Kiaske, Robert, *Crystals of Life: The Story of Salt*, Doubleday, 1968.

Stamler, Jeremiah, *et al.*, eds., *The Epidemiology of Hypertension*, Grune & Stratton, 1967.

Articles

FDA Consumer, selected issues.

Klumb, George H., "Sodium: Friend or Foe?" *Water Conditioning*, November 1975.

Light, Larry, "House Bill Would Require Food Processors to Label Sodium Content of Food," *Congressional Quarterly Weekly Report*, Oct. 17, 1981.

Nutrition Action, selected issues.

"Sodium Research Made Top Priority," *Food Engineering*, October 1981.

Stein, Jane, "Warning About Salt — Will Voluntary Labeling do the Job Without a New Law?" *National Journal*, Oct. 17, 1981.

Young, Gordon, "The Essence of Life: Salt," *National Geographic*, September 1977.

Report and Studies

Editorial Research Reports: "Food Additives," 1978 Vol. I, p. 341.

Federation of American Societies for Experimental Biology, Life Sciences Research Office, "Evaluation of the Health Aspects of Sodium Chloride and Potassium Chloride as Food Ingredients," 1979.

Levy, Phil, "Salt: Walking the Briny Line," Talking Food Co., 1976.

National Academy of Sciences, Food and Nutrition Board, "Toward Healthful Diets," 1980.

Salt Institute, "Salt Tidbits: Some Answers on Salt," 1979; "Facts About Salt: History, Production, Uses," 1980.

U.S. Department of Agriculture, "The Sodium Content of Your Food," August 1980.

U.S. Food and Drug Administration, Bureau of Foods, "Sodium in Processed Foods," June 30, 1981.

U.S. House of Representatives, Committee on Science and Technology, Subcommittee on Investigations and Oversight, "Sodium in Food and High Blood Pressure," September 1981.

Cover by Staff Artist Robert Redding

SLEEP RESEARCH

by

Jean Rosenblatt

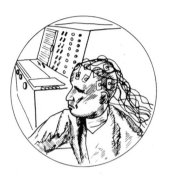

**Aug. 21
1 9 8 1**

SLEEP RESEARCH

MOST of us sleep at least once a day and wake up feeling relatively refreshed. Slipping into the unconsciousness of sleep is, for many, as natural and pleasurable as eating or laughing. But for millions of Americans, sleeping is a problem that disrupts their lives to some degree.[1] They have trouble falling asleep, they sleep too much, they fall asleep suddenly at inappropriate times, or they sporadically stop breathing during sleep. Researchers here and abroad are probing sleep's mysteries and learning how to apply their findings to help those suffering from the sleep disorders that now make up an entire area of clinical medicine.

The discovery of rapid eye movement (REM) sleep and its significance in 1953 by Dr. William C. Dement of the Stanford University Medical School marked the beginning of modern sleep research. As the understanding of normal sleep grew, researchers began to realize the potential value of evaluating abnormal or disrupted sleep. A recent trend has been the development of sleep centers that specialize in clinical studies in both the laboratory and an outpatient setting, where patients' sleep disorders are evaluated and diagnosed. When researchers discover the causes of a sleep problem, they generally send patients back to their physicians for long-term care.[2]

One does not have to be a scientist to know that to function normally, it is necessary to sleep. Yet although researchers are continually making new discoveries about the nature of sleep and what it does, they still are puzzled about exactly why people sleep. It may be that sleep evolved as organisms were adjusting to the 24-hour rotation of the Earth and that the rest phase in primitive organisms' biological rhythms gradually developed into sleep. One theory is that sleep is a physical restorative and another is that it is a kind of behavioral adaptation. "Perhaps," wrote Dr. Dement in *Some Must Watch While Some Must Sleep*, "family life itself originated from the need to sleep and to cluster for protection while in this [vulnerable] state."

Experiments in sleep deprivation have not revealed the essen-

---

[1] Estimates by sleep researchers run as high as 50 million.
[2] There are about 50 sleep clinics in the United States. To obtain a complete list, write to the Association of Sleep Disorders Centers, Stanford University Medical School, Stanford, Calif. 94305.

tial function of sleep. Prolonged loss of sleep causes disorientation and fatigue, but the effects are only temporary. "There's no evidence that sleeping poorly causes illness or death," claims Dr. Elliot Weitzman of New York's Montefiore Hospital and Medical Center.[3] Most researchers also doubt whether sleep recharges energy lost during the day, since people kept awake three to 10 days seem to need only 11 to 16 hours of sleep to catch up.

Although most people feel best when they get between seven and nine hours of sleep each night, some require less sleep and some more. Dr. Ernest Hartmann, professor of psychiatry at Tufts University School of Medicine and director of the sleep research laboratory at Boston's West-Ros-Park Mental Health Center, finds different personality traits in "short" and "long" sleepers. Short sleepers, those who sleep less than six hours, tend to be more efficient, hardworking, conformist and less creative than long sleepers, who sleep more than nine hours. Napoleon was said to have been a short sleeper and Einstein a long one.

It is common for people to need more sleep than normal during times of stress, depression or increased mental activity. Sleep needs also vary with age. Babies average about 16 hours of sleep a day. By age 3, sleep time goes down to about 12 hours and by age 5 to 11 hours, without naps. Starting in their teens, most people set a pattern of about seven and a half hours. But after 50, the amount of actual sleep decreases, though the time spent in bed may increase.

Two Kinds of Sleep and Their Cycles

We experience three distinct states of existence within a 24-hour day: (1) wakefulness, (2) dreaming or active sleep — characterized by rapid eye movements — and (3) quiet, non-dreaming sleep, or NREM (pronounced non-REM) sleep. REM sleep is as different from NREM sleep as it is from wakefulness. NREM sleep occurs in four stages and alternates with REM sleep throughout the night. In NREM sleep, breathing is slow and regular; the brain registers slow, regular activity; and the body is quiet. The body is not paralyzed, however; its senses are simply not communicating with the brain. When a person rolls over during NREM sleep, for example, he is probably awake momentarily, though unresponsive. It is during NREM sleep that people snore.

As a person falls asleep, his blood pressure, heart and breathing rates, and body temperature begin to drop. The sleeper descends through four stages of NREM sleep, becoming

---

[3] Quoted in "The Mystery of Sleep," *Newsweek*, July 13, 1981, p. 49.

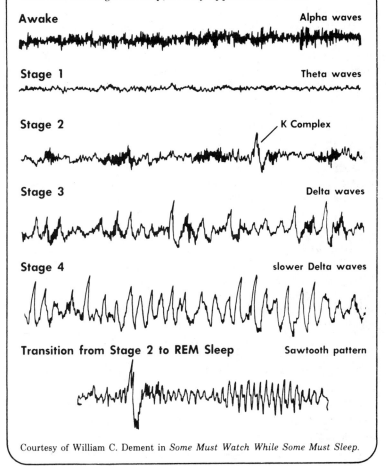

Electrical activity of the brain, eyes and muscles are recorded on an instrument called a polygraph. It monitors all three simultaneously by electrodes attached to the sleeper's scalp and face. They convey electrical impulses to the polygraph, where pens move up and down recording these signals on moving paper, which produces a pattern of waves. This record is an electroencephalogram (EEG). Wakefulness and the stages of sleep, as they appear on an EEG:

Awake   Alpha waves

Stage 1   Theta waves

Stage 2   K Complex

Stage 3   Delta waves

Stage 4   slower Delta waves

Transition from Stage 2 to REM Sleep   Sawtooth pattern

Courtesy of William C. Dement in *Some Must Watch While Some Must Sleep.*

progressively more remote from his environment and more difficult to arouse. The four sleep stages are characterized by different EEG (electroencephalogram) patterns. In the first stage, the alpha brain waves of wakefulness give way to slower theta waves and the eyes roll slowly from side to side. The exact onset of sleep is impossible to determine, even from reading an EEG. Essentially, it is the loss of awareness that distinguishes sleep from wakefulness.

After about five minutes in the twilight state of stage one, the sleeper descends to stage 2. In this stage the eyes are still, heart and breathing rates slow down further, and the EEG pattern shows spindles and K complexes. These two wave patterns appear only in NREM sleep and characterize stage 2. After several minutes the slow delta waves of stage 3 show up on the EEG, and the heart and breathing rates continue to drop.

The predominance of delta waves after about 10 minutes marks stage 4. In this stage, heart and breathing rates are about 20 to 30 percent below those in wakefulness. Anyone in this stage is extremely hard to awaken. It is in stage 4 that children begin to talk and walk in their sleep and wet their beds. The amount of stage 4 sleep is highest in infancy and decreases with age.

Thirty or forty minutes after the onset of sleep, the sleeper begins ascending back up through the stages of NREM sleep. Seventy or eighty minutes after the onset of sleep, the EEG pattern of stage 1 reappears with sawtooth waves, marking the first of several periods of REM sleep that will occur throughout the night. Almost all dreaming occurs in REM sleep.

In this state, the brain and automatic nervous system are extremely active. The sleeper's face and fingertips twitch, he stops snoring, and his breathing and heartbeat become irregular. The brain temperature soars, and the eyes dart back and forth underneath the eyelids. If a sleeper's eyelids are pulled back, he appears to be looking at something. Contractions of the middle-ear muscles also occur, although the body's large muscles in the legs, arms and trunk are completely paralyzed. If it were not for this paralysis, researchers speculate, sleepers would probably wake themselves up by thrashing around. Newborn as well as adult males also experience erections during REM sleep.[4]

The repetitive sleep cycles occur throughout the night. Each cycle varies from 70 to 110 minutes, although the average combined NREM-REM cycle is about 90 minutes. NREM sleep, especially stages 3 and 4, dominate the early part of sleep, but REM periods become progressively longer during the night, starting out at about 10 minutes and eventually lasting sometimes as long as an hour.

Biological Clock Set for 25-Hour Day

Some of the most important work in sleep research is being done in the context of circadian rhythms. Just as the tides, seasons and planets follow their own rhythmic course, the hu-

---

[4] The presence of a predictable REM-related cycle of what is known as nocturnal penile tumescence (NPT) is used to diagnose the causes of impotence. If full erection occurs during REM sleep, the cause of impotence is psychological. If NPT is weak or absent, the patient's impotence results from a physical problem.

man body is ruled by biological rhythms that govern sleeping, waking and mood swings. These are called circadian rhythms — from the Latin *circa* (about) and *dies* (day) — because they occur in periods of about 24 hours. The rhythm of sleeping and waking is usually dictated by the 24-hour rotation of the Earth around the sun.

However, when subjects at West Germany's Max Planck Institute were isolated from all time cues such as sunlight and clocks, they tended to sleep every 25 hours. This indicated that when allowed to follow innate circadian rhythms, free from environmental signals, the human body follows a 25-hour day. It has also been found that circadian rhythms may be speeded up or slowed down by an hour or two, but no more.

"[Sleep] covers a man all over, thoughts and all, like a cloak; 'tis meat for the hungry, drink for the thirsty, heat for the cold, and cold for the hot. 'Tis the current coin that purchases all the pleasures of the world cheap; and the balance that sets the king and shepherd, the fool and wise man even."

Cervantes, *Don Quixote*

Sleepiness may often result not so much from lost sleep but from a shift in circadian rhythms. This phenomenon explains, among other things, Monday morning blues and jet lag. On weekends, people generally stay up later than during the week. Their sleep and wake-up times follow more closely their natural 25-hour sleep rhythm. But on Sunday night they try to switch to the conventional 24-hour day, and suffer the results Monday morning. Swift air travel through several time zones throws the body's time out of synch with clock time, causing the fatigue and disorientation known as jet lag.

Researchers have found that a key variable in determining when, how long and how well people sleep is body temperature. Apparently sleep patterns coincide with the daily rise and fall of body temperature. The normal time for waking occurs when body temperature climbs from its low point in the early hours of the morning to its daily high at midday. When the body temperature is dropping to its lowest level, the inclination to sleep is greatest. "Our ability to go to sleep depends on when we try to do it," said Dr. Charles Czeisler of Harvard University. "If we go to sleep at the wrong time in our body's temperature cycle, we won't be able to, or we will have inefficient, fitful sleep."[5]

People are also most inept when their body temperature is at its lowest. Performance tests taken in the middle of the night show lower scores than when completed at midday. Evidence that sleep loss may not be as significant as the timing of sleep is the fact that scores are higher at noon after 24 hours of sleep deprivation than they are at 4 a.m. after only 6 hours of sleep loss. The body is ordinarily at its lowest ebb at 4 a.m., so it is not surprising that many people die in their sleep when they are physically most vulnerable.

Advances in Recent Years

NATHANIEL Kleitman, Dement's former professor at the University of Chicago, began reporting on the effects of prolonged sleep loss in humans as early as 1923. It had also been known as early as 1875 that the brain gives out electrical signals during sleep. In 1929, the electrical activity of the human brain was recorded for the first time by German scientist Hans Berger, who called this recording an electroencephalogram (EEG). Berger was the first to notice that the brain waves changed with changes in alertness.

In 1937, A. L. Loomis, E. N. Harvey and G. A. Hobart discovered from all-night EEG recordings that sleep consists of a series of recurring stages, apparently resulting from "internal stimuli." Twelve years later an Italian and an American, Giuseppe Moruzzi and Horace Magoun, working together at the Northwestern University School of Medicine, showed that stimulating a part of the brain produced "behavioral arousal" and the EEG waves of the waking state. That sleep and waking could be studied by manipulating the brain connected sleep to neurophysiology, the science of the nervous system.

Soon after these findings were reported, Eugene Aserinsky, a physiology student in Dr. Kleitman's laboratory, noticed irregular eye movements in his sleeping child. Observing sleeping adults, Aserinsky and Kleitman noticed that jerky, rapid eye movements occurred in clusters at regular intervals. Since changes in heartbeat and breathing accompanied the eye movements, Kleitman wondered whether they indicated emotional disturbance, such as dreaming. When the sleepers were awak-

---

[5] Quoted in *The Washington Post*, Dec. 11, 1980.

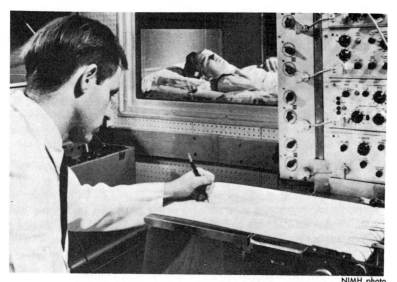

EEG Monitoring at National Institute of Mental Health

ened after the occurrence of the eye movements, they almost always reported having had dreams.

William C. Dement, at the time a second-year medical student, began recording breathing and heart rates along with brain waves during sleep. He established what the observations of others had anticipated — that sleep involves the entire body as well as the brain and that it is composed of two entirely different modes of consciousness. It was also clear to him that rapid eye movements indicated dreaming. It was once believed that the eye movements were the scanning of dream pictures by the dreamer. In fact, however, rapid eye movements and dreams originate from different parts of the brain.

At the time the relationship between REM and dreaming was confirmed, interest in sleep and dreams was high. Freudian psychoanalysis, which was based largely on Sigmund Freud's *The Interpretation of Dreams* (1900), was becoming increasingly popular, and dreams were cherished as nothing less than a possible key to the human psyche. It was also learned in the 1950s that sleep deprivation was being used to torture and extract confessions from American prisoners in the Korean War.

Dement began experimenting with REM-sleep deprivation to see if people could function normally if they were not permitted to dream. He found that the more often he tried to suppress REM sleep — by waking sleepers just as they entered this state — the more often they attempted to dream. When they were not allowed to dream, they became anxious and irritable.

That the body insists on having dreaming sleep means that REM sleep is meaningful, not "just idling," according to Dr.

149

Allan Hobson, a leading sleep researcher at the Massachusetts Mental Health Center in Boston. But if REM sleep is not a waste of time, what is it? "That's the biological riddle of my life," Dement told Editorial Research Reports. Adults usually spend about a quarter of their sleeping time — one and a half to two hours — in REM sleep. Newborn babies, on the other hand, spend about half of the time they are asleep in the REM state, and premature infants spend even more, 75 percent.

"This finding suggests," wrote Dement, "that there is a phase in the early intrauterine life of the child when REM sleep is the all-encompassing mode of existence."[6] The high percentage of REM sleep in human infants and other newborn mammals has led Dement and others to believe that this kind of sleep may be necessary for pre- and postnatal brain maturation. The essential function of REM sleep in adults, however, remains a mystery.

A Neurophysiological Dream Theory

Dreams are the bizarre, subterranean world of images we enter several times a night. Where do they come from and what do they mean? Every culture has its own unique relationship to the dream and its own version of shaman or seer to reveal the dream to the dreamer or the dreamer to himself. Sigmund Freud was one of the first scientists to explore the meaning of dreams. He theorized, in the words of science writer Margaret C. McDonald, that "dreams are the conscious expression, albeit in symbolic or disguised form, of unconscious fantasies that are repressed during the waking state."[7]

This psychological theory went virtually unchallenged until 1977, when Drs. Allan Hobson and Robert McCarley of the Massachusetts Mental Health Center and Harvard University proposed that dream content is determined by more or less random firings of nerve cells, or neurons, that occur in the brain stem during REM sleep. Higher brain centers then interpret these firings and synthesize them into a story. "The structure of the dream," McCarley wrote, "is determined not only by where the neuronal activity is going on, but also by its timing and sequence as well as its duration and intensity."[8]

The brain stem, the lowest section of the brain lying beneath the base of the skull, controls sleep and waking as well as respiration, heart rate and temperature regulation. The middle part of the brain stem is called the pons and seems to control the sleep cycle. In the pontine area are giant cells with projections going up and down the brain stem. Cells in this area,

[6] William C. Dement, *Some Must Watch While Some Must Sleep* (1974), p. 30.
[7] Margaret C. McDonald, "The Dream Debate: Freud vs. Neurophysiology," *Science News,* June 13, 1981, p. 378.
[8] Robert W. McCarley, "Where Dreams Come From: A New Theory," *Psychology Today,* December 1978.

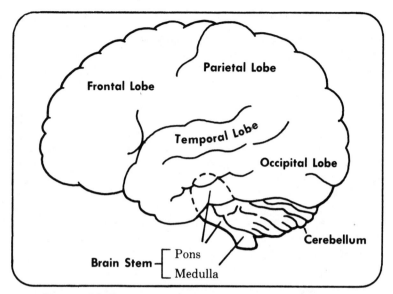

Frontal Lobe

Parietal Lobe

Temporal Lobe

Occipital Lobe

Cerebellum

Brain Stem — Pons
Medulla

according to McCarley, show increased activity before a REM period begins and reach peak activity during REM sleep. These and other findings led McCarley and Hobson to believe that the giant cells might trigger some of the activity in REM sleep.

The two scientists say that even though dreams are part of the brain's natural activity during REM sleep rather than the mind's unconscious efforts to disguise wishes and fantasies, dreams do reveal the dreamer's emotions and motivations. But these elements do not generate dreams. For example, a man's "dream about sex might be stimulated by the erection itself — or by the activation of the neural centers controlling erection" rather than by an initial sexual desire or fantasy.

McCarley and Hobson's dream model, which they call activation-synthesis, has generated heated debate among psychiatrists and psychoanalysts. Many of them believe that the theory is only speculation, and they question its applicability to psychoanalytic theory. Ramon Greenberg, a Boston psychoanalyst who has done extensive research on dreaming and learning, is one who disagrees with McCarley and Hobson's explanation of dream content. "Dreaming," said Dr. Greenberg, "seems to be a process in which the dreamer struggles to make sense of and thereby master his life experiences, while maintaining a continuing sense of himself in relation to the world. It . . . is an accurate portrayal of life as the dreamer experiences it."[9]

Depression and Sleep Cycles: A Link

Sleep researchers have found a correlation between REM sleep, circadian rhythms and mental depression. They report

---

[9] Ramon Greenberg and Chester Pearlman, "The Private Language of the Dream," in J. Natterson, ed., *The Dream in Clinical Practice* (1980), p. 95.

that depressed people have relatively more REM sleep earlier in the night and they go into the REM period much sooner than others do. These sleep abnormalities suggest that the mechanism that regulates the sleep cycle in depressives is out of phase.

Psychiatrist Gerald W. Vogel with a research team at the Georgia Mental Health Institute compared the results of REM sleep deprivation among depressed and non-depressed persons. Deprivation seemed to improve the depression, at least temporarily. The researchers concluded that the frequent awakenings necessary to arouse persons from REM sleep served to repair their irregular sleep-wake cycle. Vogel's study also supported the belief that anti-depressant drugs improve depression by reducing REM sleep.[10]

At the National Institute of Mental Health in Rockville, Md., psychiatrists Thomas Wehr and Frederick Goodwin deprived a manic-depressive volunteer of sleep for one night and then twice successively advanced her normal bedtime by six hours, thereby also advancing her wake-up time by six hours. With each advance the woman experienced relief from her depression. A third sleep phase advance had no effect, presumably because it brought her sleep schedule close to her original cycle.[11] Similar experiments have been conducted with the same results. This procedure, Dr. Wehr told Editorial Research Reports, "tends to support the idea that some abnormality in the timing of the biological clock is playing an important role in the causes of some kinds of depression."

As a treatment, advancing the sleep-wake schedule to correspond to a depressive's internal clock would not be practical. The new sleeping hours would be inappropriate, and continually advancing the sleep-wake cycle eventually re-establishes the original abnormality. When the subjects are in "a kind of therapeutic jet lag" — their biological clocks haven't adjusted to their changed hours of sleep — "that's when they are made the most nearly normal," Dr. Wehr said.

There may be a more practical way to alter the timing of depressives' circadian sleep rhythms. The two major classes of anti-depressant drugs, monoamine oxidase inhibitors and tricyclics, have been found to delay the sleep-wake cycle of experimental animals. It may be that these drugs delay the biological clocks set abnormally early in depressed people. But anti-depressants take two to three weeks to become effective, a disadvantage when there is the possibility of suicide. One way to

---

[10] See Gerald W. Vogel and others, "Improvement of Depression by REM Sleep Deprivation," *Archives of General Psychiatry*, March 1980, p. 247.
[11] See "Speeding Up the Depressive Night of the Soul," *Psychology Today*, March 1979, p. 23.

overcome this drawback is to manipulate sleep in combination with drug-taking. Sleep manipulation works immediately but is temporary, while drugs take a long time to work but have a more lasting effect.

Disorders and Treatment

I N A national survey of physicians reported in *Journal of the American Medical Association*, they estimated that more than one out of four of their patients complained of poor sleep.[12] Although patients consistently exaggerate their sleeplessness, insomnia is still the most prevalent of all sleep disorders. Insomnia sufferers have difficulty falling or remaining asleep, or else wake up too early. Chronic insomniacs generally get less of the deep (stage 4) sleep and have higher temperatures and heart rates and more body movements during sleep than is normal.

The causes of persistent insomnia are varied. They include physical conditions such as arthritis and breathing difficulties; psychological states such as depression, anxiety and stress; drugs, alcohol, caffeine and nicotine; and circadian rhythm disturbances. Most often insomnia is associated with psychological problems. "Insomniac patients often have difficulty expressing and controlling their aggressive feelings," according to Dr. Anthony Kales, director of the sleep research and treatment center at the Pennsylvania State University Medical Center. "Going to sleep represents a loss of control, and insomnia is a defense against this fear."[13]

Repressing and denying emotions and conflicts lead to emotional — hence physiological — arousal at night, resulting in sleeplessness. Eventually insomniacs begin to fear sleeplessness and then come to expect it. The result is a vicious circle of sleeplessness, fear of it, psychological conflict, physiological arousal and further sleeplessness. Dealing with the conflicts underlying insomnia through psychotherapy often relieves the sleeplessness.

Physicians report that the elderly, especially women, most frequently complain of insomnia. According to Dr. Dement, 99 percent of the elderly have disturbed sleep. Much of their sleep loss is a natural result of aging and the pain and discomfort that accompany declining health. Older people are also likely to become anxious or depressed about their physical limitations and about death.

---

[12] The survey results were reported by Joyce D. Kales and others in "Resource for Managing Sleep Disorders," *Journal of the American Medical Association*, June 1, 1979, p. 2413.

[13] Writing in the *American Handbook of Psychiatry*, Vol. 7 1981, p. 428; S. Arieti, ed.

Fear of death becomes magnified at night; even before the advent of psychoanalysis, sleep was perceived as a deathlike state, and research suggests that difficulty in falling asleep is strongly related to preoccupation with death. Drs. Richard Carrera, a psychologist at the University of Miami, and Jeffrey Elenewski, a clinical psychologist in private practice in Coral Gables, Fla., have reported on their efforts to reduce sleep-onset insomnia (the type in which it takes a long time to fall asleep) by lessening fear of death through a technique called implosive therapy.[14]

For example, the therapist might have patients imagine that they had died of an unknown disease and were buried. He continues the fantasy by having them wake up in their coffins, try to escape and then die once more. By recreating the fantasy several times, the patients become desensitized to their fear of death. They reported an immediate lessening of anxiety and after about a month, a decrease in the length of time they took to fall asleep.

A commonly recommended therapy for insomnia is relaxation training, including hatha yoga, various forms of meditation and biofeedback. These techniques seem to work best with stimulus control, a behavior modification technique developed by Dr. Richard Bootzin of Northwestern University.

Stimulus control restructures bedtime rituals and habits that interfere with sleep. Bootzin instructs insomniacs to go to bed only when sleepy and use the bed only for sleep and sexual activity — not for reading, watching television, eating or worrying. He advises them to get out of bed if they don't fall asleep within 10 minutes, to get up at the same time each day regardless of how much they slept the night before and to avoid naps during the day.[15] Experts advise troubled sleepers to avoid vigorous evening exercise and evening consumption of caffeine and alcohol. While these and stimulus control techniques may work for some insomniacs, many need counseling and supervised treatment.

Hypnotics Ineffective, Overprescribed

Researchers are finding that sleeping pills, for which over 25 million prescriptions are written each year in the United States, may actually produce sleeplessness. After about two weeks, sleeping pills, or hypnotics, become ineffective and with continued use cause frequent awakenings.[16] "In a sense, there's no

[14] Carrera and Elenewski, "Implosive Therapy as a Treatment for Insomnia," *Journal of Clinical Psychology,* June 1980, pp. 729-734.

[15] Richard R. Bootzin and Perry M. Nicassio, "Behavioral Treatments for Insomnia," in M. Herson and others, eds., *Progress in Behavior Modification,* Vol. 6, Academic Press, 1978.

[16] It has also been shown that alcohol, except in the smallest amounts, disrupts the sleep cycle, shortens REM sleep and causes frequent awakenings.

Project Sleep

Concern about sleeping pill overdoses, mental health, and the diagnosis and treatment of sleep disorders led to the formation of Project Sleep by the U.S. surgeon general a year and a half ago. Funded for three years, Project Sleep seeks to (1) develop a model curriculum and educational materials for medical schools and continuing medical education, (2) educate the public about how to recognize sleep disorders and what to do about them, and (3) stimulate and support research.

A group of 18 private organizations — including the American Medical Association, the American Automobile Association, psychologists, insurance companies, pharmacists, drug manufacturers and consumer groups — formed a coordinating council to help plan and implement Project Sleep's activities. The AAA, for example, makes available material prepared by Project Sleep on narcolepsy and excessive daytime sleepiness, which may affect driving. Information may be obtained by writing Project Sleep ADAMHA, Room 17-60, 5600 Fishers Lane, Rockville, Md. 20857.

such thing as a sleeping pill," said Dr. Charles Pollak of the Sleep-Wake Disorders Center at Montefiore Hospital. "All we can do is impair people's ability to be awake, and there's no evidence people are better off in their daytime lives for having slept with medication."[17]

Although the effectiveness of most pills begins decreasing after about a week, refill prescriptions are casually granted. A government-sponsored study in 1979 concluded that up to two million Americans take pills every night for more than two months at a time and that more than eight million use sleeping pills in a year.[18] Many people who take hypnotics habitually do so to avoid withdrawal symptoms that result from a rapid or sudden discontinuance of the medication. These symptoms include disturbed sleep and sleep loss.

The two major classes of sleeping pills are barbiturates and the more frequently used benzodiazepines. The most obvious danger of barbiturates is that they are heavily addictive and in relatively small doses can cause coma or death. The benzodiazepines, which include Valium and Librium, may be even riskier. When combined with alcohol, they can also cause death. The most common drug of this class is flurazepam, which under the trade name Dalmane accounts for more than half of all sleeping pill prescriptions.

---

[17] Quoted in *Newsweek,* July 13, 1981, p. 51.
[18] The study, "Sleeping Pills, Insomnia, and Medical Practice," was conducted by the Institute of Medicine-National Academy of Sciences and was written by a panel headed by William G. Anlyan, vice president for health affairs at Duke University. For *Science* magazine's appraisal of the study, see its issue of April 20, 1979, p. 287.

A Natural Sleeping Pill

A glass of milk before bedtime actually helps some people sleep. Milk and certain other protein foods contain L-tryptophan, an amino acid found in the body that stimulates the production of serotonin. Serotonin is a neurotransmitter in the brain involved in generating sleep.

The strongest evidence that L-tryptophan may be a natural hypnotic comes from research done by Dr. Ernest Hartmann, director of the sleep research laboratory at the West-Ros-Park Mental Health Center in Boston. Dr. Hartmann gave L-tryptophan and placebos to several young volunteers who were not insomniacs but who said they required about half an hour to fall asleep. After they took L-tryptophan, the time decreased to about 15 minutes. They also tended to wake up fewer times in the middle of the night. However, L-tryptophan does not work for all insomniacs, subsequent tests have shown.

Dalmane is less addictive than barbiturates, and people develop a tolerance to it more slowly. But the drug remains in the body much longer. So after a week the user's system might have four to six times as much of the drug as it had the first night. Researchers have found that this drug impairs reasoning and diminishes alertness during the day and reduces hand-eye coordination, which is important for driving.

According to the government's study of sleeping pills, they "should have only a limited place in contemporary medicine" and "physicians should rarely, if ever, prescribe hypnotic drugs beyond 2 to 4 weeks." Researchers recommend that physicians learn more about insomnia and the ill effects of hypnotics and offer alternatives such as office counseling and referrals for therapy. And users of sleeping pills need to be educated, Dr. Hartmann has advised. "Whether they are considering consulting a physician about insomnia or medicating themselves with over-the-counter drugs, they should at least understand the multiple causes of insomnia and various possibilities for treatment, as well as the temporary nature of many forms of insomnia."[19]

Disturbances of the Sleep-Wake Cycle

Many who think they suffer from insomnia may actually be experiencing a "disturbed circadian sleep-wake cycle," such as those caused by jet lag or changes in their work shifts. While jet lag or work change symptoms are likely to be temporary, some other forms of sleep-cycle disorders may be persistent. People in these situations are unable to sleep for sustained periods of time, wake up before they have had a full amount of sleep, and

[19] Ernest Hartmann, "The Sleeping Pill: Do the Risks Outweigh Whatever Benefits?", *Science Digest*, March 1979, p. 75.

want to sleep when it's time to be awake. While awake they feel groggy but have trouble falling asleep at bedtime. Jet lag, though transient and a mere annoyance for vacationers, poses severe problems for airline pilots, traveling businessmen and diplomats who need to make important decisions when they normally would be sleeping. Irregular work schedules present the same kind of hazards to doctors, nurses, air-traffic controllers, policemen, firemen and long-haul truck drivers, among others.

There is also the "delayed sleep-phase syndrome." Its sufferers are the classic "night people." Typically, they are unable to fall asleep until 2 to 6 a.m. But when they are not on a strict schedule, they have no trouble sleeping. Moreover, they sleep for a normal length of time and wake up spontaneously feeling refreshed. Dr. Weitzman reports that "the use of hypnotic drugs, alcohol, behavior modification techniques, sleep hypnosis, psychotherapy and a variety of home remedies have repeatedly failed these patients."[20] In the Laboratory of Human Chronophysiology that Dr. Weitzman established at Montefiore Hospital, he uses chronotherapy to shift patients to a new sleep-wake schedule. This technique progressively delays sleep by three hours each day until the desired time for going to sleep is achieved.

Symptoms and Impact of Narcolepsy

Though troublesome, most sleep disorders are not disabling. Narcolepsy, an exception, is potentially disabling, and it is estimated to affect as many as 250,000 people in the United States. The two most disabling symptoms are excessive daytime sleepiness (EDS) and cataplexy. Narcoleptics feel sleepy and may fall asleep at inappropriate times — say, during a meal or in conversation — regardless of how much sleep they had the night before. Sometimes sleepiness occurs so suddenly that it is experienced as a sleep attack. These bouts of sleep usually last for less than 30 minutes but can continue for several hours.

Cataplexy is a sudden loss of muscle tone, usually triggered by laughter, elation, surprise, anger or some other strong emotion. A cataplectic attack might range from a partial, brief weakness of the muscles to a complete loss of muscular control. In that condition, the narcoleptic collapses and is unable to move or speak, though he may still be conscious. When cataplexy first appears, the symptoms usually are mild and infrequent. But they become more serious and occur more often

---

[20] Elliot D. Weitzman, "Sleep and Its Disorders," *Annual Review of Neuroscience,* 1981, p. 402. Dr. Weitzman also discusses his work in the draft of a chapter titled "Chronobiological Disorders: Analytical and Therapeutic Techniques" to be published in September 1982 in *Disorders of Sleeping and Waking: Indications and Techniques,* Christian Guilleminault, ed.

before reaching a maximum level that varies from person to person. The attacks last from a few seconds to 30 minutes; they may occur hundreds of times a day or as infrequently as twice a year. If the attack comes upon a person who is sitting or lying down, it sometimes turns into a sleep attack.

The educational, social and work life of narcoleptics suffer if their symptoms are other than very mild and if they have not been properly diagnosed and treated. Excessive sleepiness impairs their ability to read, study and learn. Teachers, parents and spouses "frequently and incorrectly attribute motivational concerns to the symptoms," according to William Baird, director of the American Narcolepsy Association. "For instance, a husband will complain that his wife falls asleep everytime he talks with her, or seeks some closer relationship, and he wrongly assumes that the sleepiness is a hostile gesture of rejection."[21] Because narcoleptics learn to control, to some degree, their cataleptic attacks by guarding their emotional responses, the emotional lives of narcoleptics are severely restricted.

"When I lie down I say, when shall I arise and the night be gone? And I am full of tossings to and fro until the dawning of the day."

Job 7:4

Symptoms of narcolepsy usually appear in adolescence, although it usually takes years for the symptoms to be correctly diagnosed. The disorder seems to be a lifelong one, although by middle age narcoleptics usually learn to control the emotional responses that trigger cataplexy. Still, many narcoleptics are unable to work full-time.

The causes of narcolepsy are unknown, but researchers believe the disease stems from a defect in the central nervous system. There is evidence of genetics being involved: persons related to narcoleptics are 60 times more likely than others to have narcolepsy. Stanford University researchers, observing a colony of narcoleptic dogs, have learned that narcolepsy in one breed of dogs is determined by a single gene.

---

[21] William P. Baird, "Narcolepsy: A Non-Medical Presentation," American Narcolepsy Association, 1977. The American Narcolepsy Association (Box 5846, Stanford, Calif. 94305) was formed in 1975 to help solve the problems associated with narcolepsy and related sleep disorders. The association conducts self-help group meetings for narcoleptics, identifies diagnostic facilities and physicians knowledgeable about and interested in treating narcolepsy, disseminates information to narcoleptics, physicians and the public, and encourages and supports research.

A definite diagnosis of narcolepsy can be made with a clinical sleep laboratory test. Currently, the only effective treatment consists of a combination of two drugs — amphetamines to prevent sleep attacks and anti-depressants to prevent the muscle weakness and paralysis of cataplexy. Narcoleptics are also advised to avoid liquor and take naps during the day.

Breathing Difficulties of Older People

Sleep apnea, in which breathing actually stops during sleep, is the only sleep disorder that is potentially fatal. Persons who suffer from it partially wake up when their breathing stops and then go back to sleep after they have caught their breath. In a recent study at Stanford, researchers found that the 35 people being observed stopped breathing between 68 and 682 times each night. The length of the apnea (non-breathing period) lasted between 10 and 190 seconds (3 minutes, 10 seconds).

According to Dr. Dement, full-blown sleep apnea exists in about 1 percent of the middle-aged population, and for many others of that age it is present as a borderline condition. He believes that only half of the people over age 60 breathe normally during sleep. Anyone at any time can develop sleep apnea, which is thought to be a defect of the central nervous system. Symptoms may appear gradually or suddenly. The disorder is particularly bizarre in that it can be detected only during sleep; medical examinations reveal no special physical abnormalities among its victims during their waking hours. Loud snoring is the main sign of sleep apnea, although snoring also has other causes.

There are two main kinds of sleep apnea. In central sleep apnea, the diaphragm, the muscle that helps move air in and out of the lungs, stops functioning at the onset of sleep. More common and more dangerous is upper airway sleep apnea in which there is an abnormal loss of tone in the muscles of the tongue, throat and larynx. The throat collapses, blocking air flow. The increased effort of the diaphragm working to get air in and out of the lungs eventually wakes the person up and he resumes breathing.

People who suffer from central sleep apnea usually complain of insomnia. Although they are unaware of apnea attacks, many are aware of awakening several times during the night and having trouble getting back to sleep. Those with upper airway apnea complain of excessive daytime sleepiness and are completely unaware of their disrupted sleep. They sometimes have early morning headaches and hallucinations while awake.

The daytime sleepiness of people with sleep apnea is caused by lack of oxygen at night, since the oxygen content of the blood decreases when breathing stops. Apnea attacks cause blood pressure to rise and may lead to cardiac arrest. Over time apnea can cause heart disease and chronic high blood pressure. Many persons with severe undiagnosed sleep apnea die in their sleep; it also is a cause of sudden infant death syndrome.

Although there is no known cure for sleep apnea, certain drugs can reduce the number of attacks of central sleep apnea and surgery (a tracheostomy) can reduce or eliminate upper airway apnea. A hole is made in the trachea so that air can move freely in and out of the lungs at night. During the day the hole is capped and the patient breathes normally.

A lot goes on during the third of our lives in which we remain mostly unconscious. Although sleep is less of a mystery now than it was a century ago, it still holds some secrets. Unlocking them will no doubt reveal more connections between our body and mind and our conscious and unconscious lives, and bring relief to millions seeking sleep's ease.

Selected Bibliography

Books

Arieti, S., ed., *American Handbook of Psychiatry*, Vol. 7, Basic Books, 1981.

Dement, William C., *Some Must Watch While Some Must Sleep*, W. H. Freeman, 1974.

Mendelson, Wallace B. and others, *Human Sleep and Its Disorders*, Plenum Press, 1977.

Natterson, J., ed., *The Dream in Clinical Practice*, J. Aronson, 1980.

Articles

Galvin, Ruth Mehrtens, "Probing the Mysteries of Sleep," *The Atlantic,* February 1979.

Hartmann, Ernest, "The Sleeping Pill: Do the Risks Outweigh Whatever Benefits?" *Science Digest,* March 1979.

McCarley, Robert W., "Where Dreams Come From: A New Theory," *Psychology Today,* December 1978.

McDonald, Margaret C., "The Dream Debate: Freud vs. Neurophysiology," *Science News,* June 13, 1981.

"The Mystery of Sleep," *Newsweek,* July 13, 1981.

"Speeding Up the Depressive Night of the Soul," *Psychology Today,* March 1979.

"Study Finds Sleeping Pills Overprescribed," *Science,* April 20, 1979.

Vogel, Gerald W. and others, "Improvement of Depression by REM Sleep Deprivation," *Archives of General Psychiatry,* March 1980.

Weitzman, Elliot D., "Sleep and Its Disorders," *Annual Review of Neuroscience,* 1981.

Reports and Studies

Baird, William P., "Narcolepsy: A Non-Technical Summary" and "Sleep Apnea: A Non-Technical Presentation," American Narcolepsy Association, 1977.

STRESS MANAGEMENT

by

William V. Thomas

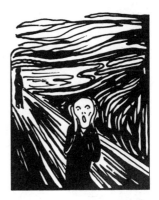

Nov. 28
1 9 8 0

STRESS MANAGEMENT

THE IMAGES of stress are everywhere: people pushing and shoving to get a seat on the commuter bus; office managers tearing into their work and skipping lunch to make deadlines; couples arguing over money; children feeling neglected by their parents and parents feeling guilty for neglecting their children. Stress, no matter what form it takes, means pressure, uncertainty and loss of a sense of control over events. It affects job performance, social relationships and the personal well-being of millions of Americans. According to the U.S. Clearinghouse for Mental Health Information, American businesses lose $17 billion annually because of employees' stress-related disabilities. Health authorities estimate that as many as 60 percent of all doctor visits in this country are prompted by signs of psychological stress rather than a specific illness.

Psychologists have been saying for years that the Christmas season is a period of increased stress and tension. The outward signs of festivity often belie the destructive pressures that many people feel at this time. "Christmas, perhaps more than any other holiday, brings with it a whole series of pre-programmed expectations," said Dr. Thomas A. Wehr, a Washington psychiatrist. "Christmas tends to make one think about the contentment associated with childhood, about family connections and the fulfillment of hopes. But it also makes people think about loss, and the things missing from their lives. The world looks bright, much brighter, in fact, than a lot of people feel. And it's that contrast that produces stress."[1]

While there is no objective evidence proving that life in America today is any more stressful than life was in other societies of the past, many clinical researchers seem to think it is. "I doubt if the people of other times had the information overload that we have," said Dr. Daniel X. Freedman, chairman of the University of Chicago's psychiatry department.[2] Many mental health authorities believe that the demands of modern life are a primary cause of stress. "We are indeed victims of our own technology," wrote behavioral specialist Jere E. Yates. "None of us wants to give up the most luxurious style of living that man has ever known, nor do we want to turn back the

[1] Interview, Nov. 21, 1980.
[2] Quoted in *The Wall Street Journal*, April 2, 1979.

clock and give up modern conveniences such as fast planes and cars that wisk us to our destinations in minutes or hours. Yet the speed of our modern machines has caused our internal systems to speed up, moving at an ever faster pace and creating what some are now calling 'hurry sickness.' "[3]

Of course, different people have different reactions to stressful situations. For some, stress may only manifest itself as occasional periods of nervousness. For others, however, chronic stress can have harmful, even fatal, results. Everyone has some point at which excessive stress exacts a toll. And with the incidence of so-called "life-style illnesses" — cancer and heart disease — on the rise, managing stress and its unhealthy side effects looms as one of medicine's biggest challenges.

Physical and Mental Reactions to Stress

The term "stress," as it is used in engineering, describes the capacity of a structure to withstand strain. In psychology, it refers to a variety of outside pressures that affect behavior. If not excessive, stress can serve a useful purpose, such as preparing a person to meet a threat or perform a certain task. Dr. Hans Selye, recognized as the father of stress research, believes that certain kinds of stress — what he calls "eustress" — are good for people. "A game of tennis or a passionate kiss can produce considerable stress without conspicuous damage," he wrote in 1956.[4] It is when stress is severe — or when an individual has a low tolerance for pressure — that problems can occur. The high divorce rate, crime and drug use are all believed to be linked in some way to stress.[5]

Selye divides the human response to stress into three stages: (1) alarm, including a "report" to the endocrine glands; (2) resistance, with the aid of stepped-up production of adrenal hormones; and (3) exhaustion, collapse, or relaxation after a stressful assault has subsided. The psychosomatic effects of stress, however, follow no predictable pattern, and may appear in various disguises. Headaches, stomach upsets, fatigue, palpitations, and pains of all sorts can have their origin in stress. Digestive troubles in the form of nausea, constipation, diarrhea or ulcers can be stress-related. Extreme stress can produce psychological disturbances, such as depression and despair, and in some cases may even lead to suicide.

People develop certain adaptive reactions to prolonged stress. But Selye warns that over a period of time these reactions can wear down the body's physical and emotional defenses,

---

[3] Jere E. Yates, *Managing Stress: A Businessperson's Guide* (1979), pp. 3-4. Yates is a professor of organizational behavior and management at Pepperdine University in Malibu, Calif.

[4] Hans Selye, *The Stress of Life* (1956), p. 53. Selye is professor emeritus at McGill University in Montreal, Canada.

[5] See "Stress in Modern Life," *E.R.R.*, 1970 Vol. II, pp. 527-542.

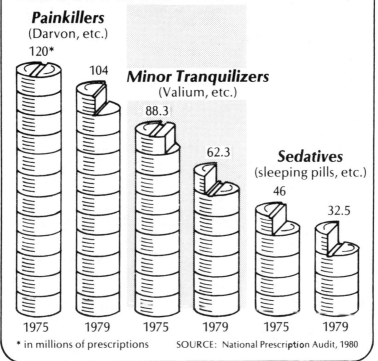

Decline in Prescription Drug Use

The use of tranquilizers and other nerve-calming prescription drugs is on the decline, according to recent statistics compiled by the National Prescription Audit, a private drug survey organization. Authorities say the drop suggests that doctors are exercising more caution in prescribing drugs for their patients and patients are becoming more aware of the potential hazards involved in drug use. Legally filled prescriptions fell from 88.3 million in 1975 to 62.3 million in 1979.

Painkillers
(Darvon, etc.)
120*
104

Minor Tranquilizers
(Valium, etc.)
88.3
62.3

Sedatives
(sleeping pills, etc.)
46
32.5

1975   1979   1975   1979   1975   1979

* in millions of prescriptions   SOURCE: National Prescription Audit, 1980

exposing it to serious illness. "Our reserves of adaptation energy could be compared to an inherited fortune from which we can make withdrawals," he wrote in *Stress Without Distress* (1974). "But there is no proof that we can also make additional deposits. We can squander our adaptability recklessly, 'burning our candle at both ends,' or we can learn to make this valuable resource last long, by using it wisely and sparingly, only for the things that are worthwhile and cause the least distress." Selye's notion about the conservation of adaptive energy is only hypothesis. However, his basic assumption that stress weakens the body's vital organs has been borne out by others.

'Type A' Personality and Heart Disease

In 1974, two cardiologists, Meyer Friedman and Ray H.

Rosenman, published evidence of increased coronary disease in people who exhibited what they called "Type A" behavior. The Type A personality, as they described it in a popular book on the subject, is marked by a high degree of competitiveness, impatience, frustration and anger. Friedman and Rosenman estimated that roughly half the adults in the United States were Type A personalities.

The Type A individual, Friedman and Rosenman found, is forever in a hurry. Not only is he obsessed with the need to accomplish something, to be engaged in some activity he considers worthwhile, he must not waste a single minute in the process. Time is the Type A person's chief enemy, and he is always trying to beat the clock by setting unrealistic deadlines. When he is not putting pressure on himself to complete tasks on time, he is punishing himself with guilt whenever he is late — which he frequently is since he tends to schedule more activities than he can finish.

Closely related to the Type A individual's preoccupation with time is his urge to judge the results of his work in quantitative terms. Type A's generally see themselves as successful people, but they are nearly always under stress. It is stress, however, largely of their own making. Type A personalities are never satisfied with what they have achieved. Accordingly, their penchant for self-measurement makes them victims of an endless exercise in futility.

People who fall into what Friedman and Rosenman labeled the "Type B" behavior pattern are much more easygoing. Relatively free of the sense of urgency that drives the Type A person, the Type B individual can relax without feeling guilt-ridden. He seems to derive a healthy incentive from competition without being totally absorbed by the struggle to succeed.

Type A behavior is common in the United States because our industrialized society encourages and rewards it. The hard-driving, achievement-oriented employee usually is considered an asset in most organizations. However, the price this person often pays is a greater risk of heart disease and other related coronary problems. In *Type A Behavior and Your Heart* (1974), Friedman and Rosenman concluded that "subjects severely afflicted with [the Type A] behavior pattern exhibited every blood fat and hormone abnormality that the majority of coronary patients also showed. In other words, the same blood abnormalities that so many of our colleagues believe precede and possibly bring on coronary heart disease were already present in our Type A subjects. . . . The logic is irresistable: the behavior pattern itself gives rise to the abnormalities." Cardiovascular diseases kill more than a million Americans each year, according to the National Center for Health Statistics, and are responsible for 37.8 percent of the deaths in this country, annually.[6]

While those with Type A personalities seem particularly vulnerable to stress-related illnesses, other people have psychological qualities that seem to make them particularly resilient. Two researchers at the University of Chicago, Suzanne C. Kobasa and Salvatore R. Maddi, have defined some of the characteristics of what they call "hardiness." Stress-resistant people, they said, have a specific set of attitudes toward life — an openness to change, a feeling of involvement in whatever they are doing and a sense of control over their lives. Those who possess these qualities, the researchers found, are much less vulnerable to such stress-related illnesses as ulcers, colitis, hypertension and heart disease. "The mechanism whereby stressful life events produce illness is presumably physiological," Kobasa said. "Yet whatever this physiological response is, the personality characteristics of hardiness may cut into it, decreasing the likelihood of breakdown into illness."[7] A two-year study of 259 business executives conducted by Kobasa and Maddi indicated that a "hardy" personality might "decrease your chance of being ill by 50 percent."

On-the-Job Pressures; Executive Health

Perhaps the most damaging consequences of stress are found in the business world, where its day-to-day effects on executives as well as average workers can result in poor performance, absenteeism, low productivity, industrial sabotage and death. In a recent study of on-the-job stress, behavioral specialists Ari Kiev and Vera Kohn found that the most stress-producing factors at work are the pressures to perform a job well, time limitations, the disparity between an employee's or manager's own goals and the expectations of the organization, the political climate of an organization and the lack of feedback on work performance.[8]

Job pressures affect everyone from the poor worker, for whom job security is the most important source of worry, to women entering or re-entering the job market. For decades, businesses have recognized the problems caused by stress, but only in the last several years have they begun to invest large sums of money in stress management. Companies have responded to the stress-induced problems of their employees by attempting to improve working conditions, providing more vacations and

---

[6] Figures for 1977, the latest year for which statistics are available.
[7] Quoted by Maya Pines in "Psychological Hardiness," *Psychology Today,* December 1980, p. 36.
[8] Ari Kiev and Vera Kohn, "Executive Stress," American Management Associations, 1979, p. 2.

sick leave, and adding medical and psychological counseling staffs. Some corporations have also set up special stress management programs for their employees. These often include fitness training, meditation lessons and biofeedback clinics.[9] According to the American Association of Fitness Directors in Business and Industry, more than 750 corporations and businesses had cardiovascular fitness programs in 1978.

Because of the uniqueness of stress patterns and the diversity of the events that elicit them, one approach that is gaining wide popularity is individualized stress management training for business executives. In fact, in the last decade, executive health has become an industry of its own, with hundreds of large and small psychological service centers opening across the country. One such company, Executive Health Examiners of New York City, advertises itself this way: "The value of an 'ounce of prevention' . . . has long been recognized by the medical and dental professions. What is good practice for strengthening physical resources proves to be equally valuable when applied to mental resources. Periodic examinations of the way a person copes with stress can both detect and head off early problems as well as strengthen healthy mental resources." Thus businessmen and corporate executives are being sold on the idea that they should learn how to control stress before it controls them.

University of Chicago researcher Suzanne C. Kobasa believes that the new emphasis in corporations on stress management could have unexpected, negative side effects. "Unfortunately," she said, "many business corporations, in their eagerness to set up stress-management programs, gyms on their top floors and cardiac units in the medical department, seem to be buying into this negative, narrow view of stress. The executive is told that stress is harmful and that attempts will be made to reduce it; but in the meantime, use biofeedback or the exercise machine to ready your body for the assault." According to Kobasa, the executive's social group thus provides little support for the view that stress is positive or controllable.[10]

The effects of stress on women executives have received a lot of attention in recent years.[11] Because of the added burdens created by their dual responsibilities — at home and at work — some worry that women supervisors will be even more vulnerable than men to stress-related diseases. But so far there is no conclusive medical evidence to support this. In fact, a recent study indicated that professional women are less likely to develop heart disease than are women clerical workers, including

---

[9] See "Workers' Changing Expectations," *E.R.R.*, 1980 Vol. II, pp. 777-800.
[10] Quoted in *Psychology Today, op. cit.,* p. 40.
[11] See "Women in the Executive Suite," *E.R.R.*, 1980 Vol. II, pp. 485-504.

secretaries, bookkeepers, bank cashiers and sales clerks. The study also found that women as a group continue to enjoy lower rates of coronary heart disease than men and that going to work only slightly increases the risk for women.[12]

According to Chicago psychiatrist Irvin H. Gracer, women "are not as likely to suffer stress-related illnesses as men in similar jobs because they find it easier to vent their emotions and verbalize their frustration." But, he added, "if women executives attempt to emulate the emotional pattern of their male peers and restrain their tendencies to be open and candid about how they feel, they also may pay the penalty that men pay."[13]

Clinical Approaches To Stress

THE TERM "psychosomatic" first was used in 1818 by Johann C. Heinroth, a German medical researcher, to describe the physical effects of mental disturbances. But for centuries scientists had recognized the interaction of mind and body in maintaining — or disrupting — human health. William Harvey (1578-1657) was the first to note an association between mental or physical stress and the rate of pumping of blood by the heart. Another English physician, Thomas Sydenham (1624-1689), found that the root of many physical diseases "cannot be . . . brought to light by . . . an examination of the body" alone. In 1798, Philippe Pinel, practicing medicine in Paris, observed that some diseases affecting the body are emotional in origin and consequently do not show such casual signs as "inflammation or morbid alteration in structure."

Sigmund Freud, in the early years of his practice, treated a number of patients who, as a psychosomatic effect of anxiety, were paralyzed physically in some part of the body or had a sensory organ that did not function. Freud began to wonder about the machinery whereby the mind reacts to stressful experiences and churns out behavioral responses. He reached the conclusion that life's incessant frustrations are a direct cause of physical and mental illnesses.

Freud was one of the first to develop a theoretical model of what happens when an individual is subjected to stress. First, he said, there is a danger or threat. Then anxiety ensues. Finally, the individual puts into action his defenses against

[12] The results of the study were published in the February 1980 issue of the *American Journal of Public Health.*
[13] Quoted by Jane Adams in *Women on Top* (1979), p. 173.

anxiety. These defense mechanisms are avoidance, denial and repression. Central to Freud's thinking on the causes of stress was his idea that there is an irremediable antagonism between the demands of human instinct and the restrictions of civilization. The natural life of man, he believed, is one of aggression and ego self-satisfaction. But the whole structure of culture has been designed to put curbs on these impulses. The result, Freud suggested in *Civilization and Its Discontents* (1930), is an "inherited unhappiness" imposed by the community on its members. This unhappiness, he concluded, may often "reach heights that the individual finds hard to tolerate."[14]

Freudian theories had little influence in studies of stress-induced health problems before World War II. After the war, however, Freud's explanation of the emotional factors involved in physical illness gained greater currency. Certain physical disorders were conceived as the patient's way of expressing repressed guilt or hostility. One theory had it that the individual, in order to escape anxiety, regresses to an internal state of infancy after which adult physiology may break down into patterns of disease. Another theory proposed that the cumulative effect of repeated stress impairs an individual's most vulnerable organ. It is hypothesized that the physiological processes that accompany rage or fear (accelerated heart activity, secretion of adrenaline, dilation of the blood vessels, reduction of digestive activity, etc.) were nature's way of preparing primitive man for "fight or flight," but in civilized man these outlets are blocked. Some master the dilemma with psychological adjustment, while others, unable to cope effectively, may develop psychosomatic symptoms.

Search for Ways to Cope With Tension

In the 1950s, psychologists joined forces with existentialist thinkers who attributed stress and other related mental woes to the irrationality of the human condition. French philosopher Jean-Paul Sartre and other existentialists held that life is characterized by anxiety resulting from the absurdity of things, the disjunction between the human urge for sense and reason and the basically irrational nature of existence. In the absence of any pre-ordained meaning in life, Sartre believed that man is free to create his own identity by whatever he decides to do. Existential psychoanalysts tried to open up their patients' minds to this notion, believing that such understanding is a step toward dealing with stress.

The work of psychiatrists later was supplemented by both scientific and popular prescriptions for cultivating peace of

---

[14] Sigmund Freud, *Civilization and Its Discontents* (1961 ed.), p. 80.

Now What?

If stress and anxiety are often associated with the fear of failure, they also can occur as a result of success. A sense of panic frequently accompanies the fulfillment of a particular ambition. Suddenly, after accomplishing something important, a person may feel that the principal struggle in his life is over and nothing is left.

Since achievements seldom match expectations, any success might be considered a potential source of emotional letdown. "If you're unsatisfied, you're too busy grabbing and reaching out for some goal or great virtue," said psychotherapist Rollo May. "It's when your basic needs are met that you look for something more. Once you've made enough money, you're out for bigger game."

May called the problem "success ennui." It can happen to anyone. But it's especially common, he noted, among people who set high standards for themselves. May's solution was simple. Success in achieving one goal should not be seen as an end in itself but rather as an opportunity to create new objectives or to revive old ones. "Find new goals," he wrote, "that will give you a sense of enjoyment and meaning . . . a taste for adventure."

mind and relaxation as a cure for stress. During the last two decades, many people sought inner peace from life's anxieties by methods originating in the Orient. Zen Buddhism and Hindu meditation attracted those who were willing to try exercises in mental concentration as a path to stress-free living. Similar motivation prompted some to become devotees of religious cults or self-awareness groups.[15]

Group meetings for individuals who wished to improve their ability to cope with stress began after World War II when the National Training Laboratory at Bethel, Maine, organized training groups, known as "T-groups," for enhancing the human relations skills of business executives. The theory behind the "T-groups" was that they helped participants improve their organizational effectiveness. Although the worth of the "T-group" concept became the subject of debate within professional circles, it nevertheless gave rise to several important offshoots. One was the encounter group, considered by many counseling experts as the most important social invention of the century. The best known of the organizations that conduct encounter groups is the Esalen Institute at Big Sur, Calif. Established in the 1950s, the institute has treated thousands of people. A typical session may consist of both sexes, sitting naked in a shallow swimming pool. Participants might then express themselves by screaming or touching someone's face.

---

[15] See "Cults in America and Public Policy," *E.R.R.*, 1979 Vol. I, pp. 265-284.

In the early 1970s, the encounter group format was adopted by Werner Erhardt, founder of "est" (for Erhardt seminar training). Preaching a combination of existential philosophy and what some have called a kind of creative self-aggrandizement, Erhardt claimed that est sessions were effective in ridding trainees of guilt, social fears and stress. Est meetings normally involve participants spending time in isolated groups, hearing lectures and taking part in therapeutic exercises. While est has been praised by many who say it helped them gain control of their lives, critics argue that its methods as well as its results are questionable. Group leaders, they maintain, are often no more than "weekend messiahs" who conduct trainees through an intense emotional experience with little or no long-term effect.

Biofeedback Method of Fighting Stress

"All the best science has soft edges, limits that are still obscure and extend . . . into areas that are not wholly explicable," biologist Lyall Watson wrote in 1973.[16] One of those areas is the stress treatment technique known as biofeedback. Biofeedback is the name given to a process by which individuals learn to sense instantly what is going on within their bodies. Through this knowledge, they may then learn to control bodily functions that were once thought to be involuntary.

Research in this field has been going on for more than 30 years, but interest in it has greatly accelerated as hopes for medical applications have risen. Aside from being effective in the control of asthma, epilepsy, hyperkinesis (excessive motion) and other functional disorders, biofeedback has proven especially valuable in treating symptoms of stress. "Studies have shown . . . that high levels of stress can be fought . . . with a combination of techniques designed to induce control of a particular area in which stress is manifest," wrote Jere E. Yates. "Biofeedback works well on specific disorders such as high blood pressure. We don't know how people lower their blood pressure through biofeedback, but we do know that it can be done."[17]

Biofeedback involves going beyond those muscles subject to one's voluntary will to those internal processes not heretofore considered responsive to the human will. This advance was made possible by the development of electronic technology that originated in the mid-1940s. Devices were created that, when attached to a living creature, would give immediate external signals to indicate internal functions. This is the essential meaning of biofeedback: It is a "feeding back" to the subject (or

---

[16] Lyall Watson, *Supernature* (1973), p. 244.
[17] Yates, *op. cit.*, pp. 137-138.

Physical and Mental Signs of Stress

Physical Signs	Mental Signs
High blood pressure	A constant feeling of uneasiness
Excess weight for your age and height	Constant irritability with family and work associates
Lack of appetite	Boredom with life
A desire to eat as soon as a problem arises	A recurring feeling of being unable to cope with life
Frequent heartburn	Anxiety about money
Chronic diarrhea or constipation	Morbid fear of disease, especially cancer and heart disease
An inability to sleep	
A feeling of constant fatigue	Fear of death — your own and others'
Muscle spasm	
Frequent headaches	A sense of suppressed anger
Bruxism or grinding teeth	An inability to have a good laugh
Shortness of breath	
A liability to fainting or nausea	A feeling of being rejected by your family
Persistent sexual problems (frigidity, impotence, fear)	A sense of despair at being an unsuccessful parent
Excessive nervous energy which prevents sitting still or relaxing	Dread as the weekend approaches
An inability to cry or a tendency to burst into tears easily	A feeling that you cannot discuss your problems with anyone
A need for aspirin or some other medication daily	An inability to concentrate for any length of time or finish a project

Source: *Managing Stress* (1979)

in some cases to the experimenter) of information on what is happening at that moment within his or her physiological system.

The unique character of the new electronic instruments is that they give an instantaneous report that the individual can immediately recognize. This is important because in operant conditioning — as this learning process is called — the reward (in this case the biological information) must be instantaneous. The information is usually channeled through a computer and presented as a flashing light or sound signal, which may represent very subtle changes in the internal process. In essence, biofeedback machines measure how stressed or how relaxed certain parts of the body are. The machines themselves do not reduce muscle tension; rather they monitor muscle activity and supply information to the subject, who then creates any change that may occur.

Muscle tension is measured by an electromyograph (EMG). The EMG monitors the amount of tension present in whatever muscle group it is attached to. Other well-known biofeedback devices include those used to record brain wave activity (electroencepalograph or EEG machine), those that measure the electrical conductivity of the skin (galvanic skin response or GSR) and those used to measure skin temperature. The first significant triumph for biofeedback was in training animal subjects to change the rate of several internal processes. Dr. Neal Miller of Rockefeller University, a psychologist who did pioneer experiments in what he called "viseral learning," found that by applying conditioning techniques he could teach laboratory animals to speed up or slow down the rate of their heartbeat, raise or lower their blood pressure, and increase or decrease their intestinal contractions.

"Exercise is one of the very finest stress-reduction techniques you can employ. . . ."

Jere E. Yates
Managing Stress (1979)

In the late 1960s, Dr. Miller began applying his findings to human subjects. The first experiments were with volunteers who succeeded in bringing their blood pressure down or up by concentrating on producing the appropriate signal from a biofeedback machine. Miller discovered that the best results occurred when patients were able to clear their minds of all stressful thoughts. Subsequent experiments have produced guarded optimism about the therapeutic applications of biofeedback. Some have even shown that certain individuals can change their heartbeats at will.

A somewhat different technique for treating stress-related symptoms was developed by Dr. Elmer Green of the Menninger Foundation. This procedure involves raising the temperature of the hands. First, patients are given devices that indicate differences between the temperature of a finger and the forehead. Then they are instructed to induce a state of deep relaxation similar in its effect to the condition sought in yoga. It has been shown that relaxation of the finger muscles causes an increased blood flow there, which often relieves the pain of stress-caused migraine headaches by inducing blood flow away from the head. Despite the extraordinary results obtained by biofeedback, there are some drawbacks. For one thing, biofeedback machines are expensive and cumbersome. Furthermore, evidence suggests that without the machines most people are unable to duplicate long-term control over internal body functions on their own.

Everyday Coping Techniques

A MERICA has been called a nation of compulsive achievers. While many politicians lately have taken to counseling moderation as a way of life for the 1980s, large numbers of people continue the mad chase after impossible goals. But the relentless struggle for promotion and perfection is in most cases not only unreasonable but unhealthy. Physicians and psychologists agree that the majority of Americans simply do not know how to relax. As a result, stress, anxiety and accompanying physical illness are often the price they pay.

Hans Selye noted in his classic study *The Stress of Life* (1956) that relaxation is the most effective means of managing stress. But Selye added that "I have always been against the advice of physicians who would send a high-strung [person] to a long, enforced exile in some health resort, with the view of relieving him from stress by absolute inactivity." Selye and other experts on stress argue that the most beneficial forms of relaxation combine elements of activity and repose.

"Genuine relaxation gives a person's body and mind an opportunity to recuperate," wrote psychologist Gene W. Brockopp. "But it is quite different from the usual concept of relaxation; which often means drinking some liquor, reading a book or watching television. Those activities are usually diversions rather than relaxations. In such diversions, the tensions of the body may actually persist or increase." Even during sleep, Brockopp wrote, "the body and the mind frequently do not completely rest. Bodily tensions may persist throughout the night while the brain continues to be active and involved with low-level worries, planning, dreaming or mechanical association which result in our feeling tired when we arise."[18]

Stress increases various physiological indications of a body's condition, such as blood pressure and heart beat. During periods of relaxation, these and other physiological indications decrease. According to Herbert Benson of the Harvard Medical School, the body's response to relaxation is "innate." Regular, voluntary

---

[18] Gene W. Brockopp, "Re-learning the Ability to Relax," unpublished monograph.

periods of relaxation, Benson suggested, "can counterbalance and alleviate" the effects of stress.[19] Benson's technique for bringing about what he calls the "relaxation response" involves the following steps: (1) sit quietly in a comfortable position; (2) keep eyes closed; (3) relax all muscles, beginning with the feet and progressing to the face; (4) breathe through the nose and count each breath silently; (5) maintain a passive attitude and permit relaxation to occur at its own pace; (6) when distracting thoughts occur, try to ignore them by concentrating on counting each breath; (7) continue for a period of 10 to 20 minutes. When finished, sit quietly for several minutes with eyes closed and then with eyes open.

Meditation, similar to the relaxing method Benson described, is a tool for gaining mastery over the process of attention. Meditation itself entails a temporary shutdown of the brain's information screening mechanisms, which are primarily responsible for producing stress. Studies have found that meditation decreases respiratory and heart rates, increases alpha brain waves (signal of a more relaxed state), lowers blood pressure and decreases muscle tension — all changes associated with de-stressing the body. Most types of meditation involve a relaxed concentration on breathing. However, one type, called Transcendental Meditation, achieves its effect through the subject's repetition of a monosyllabic word or sound. Practitioners of "TM" say that hearing this sound, or montra, not only draws the attention away from whatever is distracting or stressful but leads the unconscious mind into new realms of awareness.

Exercise as a Stress-Reduction Method

Many people maintain that the state of mental calm produced by meditation also can be achieved through physical exercise. "Exercise is one of the very finest stress-reduction techniques you can employ...," wrote Jere E. Yates. "Of course, if you aren't careful, you can overdo it and cause the exercise to become distressful or harmful. Yet, as long as you are not overdoing the strenuous activity, it can be quite beneficial."[20]

Two of the most popular forms of exercise in America today are jogging and long-distance running. Many say that running brings them tranquility, enabling them to forget everyday troubles. Running can be a "mental exercise, a kind of ambulatory yoga," Michael Fessier Jr. explained.[21] About 35 million Ameri-

---

[19] Herbert Benson, "Your Innate Asset for Combatting Stress," *Harvard Business Review*, July-August 1974, p. 49.
[20] Yates, *op. cit.*, pp. 115-116. See also "Physical Fitness Boom," *E.R.R.*, 1978 Vol. I, pp. 261-280.
[21] Michael Fessier Jr., "Transcendental Running," *Human Behavior*, July 1976, p. 18.

cans claim to participate in the sport and, according to the President's Council on Physical Fitness and Sports, about six million are regular joggers.

No one could be happier about the growing number of people huffing and puffing their way to health and happiness than is the National Jogging Association (NJA), a non-profit educational organization in Washington, D.C. Since the association was founded in 1968, its membership has grown from 400 to about 35,000. "Jogging is a convenient and inexpensive form of exercise," NJA executive director Liz Elliott said in an interview last September, "and we want to spread the word."

The benefits of achieving cardiovascular fitness through running are numerous. In sufficient quantities, running improves the efficiency of the lungs, increases the available supply of blood for carrying oxygen to all parts of the body, lowers blood pressure, improves general muscle tone, relaxes the digestive system, extends the vascular system by creating additional blood vessels and above all, strengthens the heart. Improved cardiovascular fitness also correlates with a reduction in levels of glucose, cholesterol, triglycerides, uric acid, body fat, weight and heart rate.

In addition to improved cardiovascular fitness, there is another benefit to exercise in combating excessive stress, according to Jere E. Yates. "The rest that follows exercise is a form of forced relaxation, as your body insists upon its recovery time," he wrote. "Were you not working out at all, you might be constantly caught up in a hectic pace and never allow yourself the time for relaxation. At least exercise forces you to slow down occasionally."[22]

Calming Effects of Yoga and Hypnosis

It has long been known that accomplished devotees of yoga could undergo extraordinary feats of endurance. Yet Western science until recently paid little attention to trying to explain yoga's mysteries or exploring its applications in modern life. The feats made possible by yoga are now attributed to control over certain physiological processes of the autonomic or involuntary nervous system. Yoga exercises attempt to benefit particular areas of the body by relaxing them, which in turn calms the mind.

Yoga literally means the fusing of mind and body. To accomplish this, the varieties of yoga prescribe exercises in which the subject progresses from simpler to more complex feats and, as he does so, presumably moves to higher levels of spiritual understanding. Of course, one need not accept the tenets es-

[22] Yates, *op. cit.*, pp. 122-123.

poused by yoga mystics to take part in or benefit from yoga exercises. Those who practice yoga often claim that it brings them relief from stress, better health, more vigor and a clearer mind.[23]

Hypnosis, another ancient procedure and one that has never penetrated far beyond the periphery of medical practice in the Western world, also is being seen as a means for handling stress. An hypnotic state is not the same as sleep, but rather a condition characterized by heightened awareness and sensitivity. Popularly thought of as a "spell" cast on the subject, hypnosis to a large extent depends on the active will of the person being hypnotized.

In recent years, self-hypnosis has been used successfully in treating stress cases. Self-hypnosis has the advantage of not only inducing a deep relaxation but of enabling the individual to give himself suggestions that can help him alter his thinking and behavior in ways that diminish stress. The subject undergoing self-hypnosis can put himself into a light trance by fixing his eyes on a stationary object, breathing slowly and deliberately and repeating a word like "relax" at regular short intervals. This type of hypnotic trance is completely safe and can be ended at any moment the subject wishes.

Whereas meditation is mainly a form of deep rest, hypnosis can provide both relaxation and re-training. "Hypnotic autosuggestions," that is suggestions made by the subject, can gradually transform the way a person sees himself. Under hypnosis, an individual telling himself to be more relaxed at business meetings, for example, often imagines seeing himself that way. Thus autosuggestion is reinforced by its own imagined enactment. Although medical experts advise that self-hypnosis takes time to yield results, its effect can be dramatic. Once a person comes to accept the idea that through hypnosis he can change the manner in which he responds to stress, he is well on the way to curing himself.

Self-Help and Behavioral Modification

Because it is rooted in personality, stress in most cases can be managed by changing personal habits and attitudes that promote its effects. Meditation and exercise help to relieve stress symptoms by giving individuals a feeling of self-control they might otherwise lack. But these techniques do not really treat the causes of stress. Since the stress reaction is both a physical and emotional response to events, the most sensible way of reducing stress, most psychologists say, is for the in-

---

[23] See Kenneth R. Pelletier, *Mind As Healer, Mind as Slayer* (1977).

dividual to avoid as much as possible those conditions that bring it about.

In almost every instance, the key to effectively controlling stress is changing the pace of one's life so as to minimize physical and mental fatigue and their accompanying stress disorders. For the harried professional plagued by deadlines this might mean delegating more authority to subordinates or taking more time off to maintain or regain equanimity. For the frantic perfectionist, scaling down personal goals frequently results in a reduction of anxiety. In cases where job-related pressures are a source of stress, Ari Kiev and Vera Kohn advise that a person "should try to acquire alternative interests and satisfactions so that life is in balance between work and play. What happens off the job affects energy and interest on the job and vice versa. Success in one area can raise morale and help to balance stress in another."[24]

One method of achieving this balance is to apply the basic principles of behavioral modification. Jere E. Yates offered this suggestion: "Choose a specific behavior that you want to change, note what your current behavior is and decide on your goal. As you move toward that goal, reward yourself by indulging in some pleasure that you normally do not allow yourself. If you backslide, punish yourself by withholding the reward. . . ."[25]

If self-awareness is the highest form of understanding, then gaining that awareness and putting it to use may be the best, perhaps the only, way of dealing successfully with stress. The main point to remember, Yates concluded, is that people ultimately determine how much of an effect stress will have on them, and people ultimately decide how they will manage it.

---

[24] *Executive Stress, op. cit.,* p. 56.
[25] Yates, *op. cit.,* p. 144.

▼▼▼

Selected Bibliography

Books

Benson, Herbert, *The Relaxation Response,* William Morrow and Co., 1975.

Bloomfield, Harold H., Michael Peter Cain, Dennis T. Jaffe and Robert B. Kory, *T.M.: Discovering Inner Energy and Overcoming Stress,* Delacorte Press, 1975.

Bower, Sharon A. and Gordon H. Bower, *Asserting Your Self,* Addison-Wesley, 1976.

Friedman, Meyer and Ray H. Rosenman, *Type A Behavior and Your Heart,* Fawcett, 1974.

Goldberg, Philip, *Executive Health,* McGraw-Hill, 1978.

Karlins, Marvin and Lewis M. Andrews, *Biofeedback: Turning on the Power of Your Mind,* Warner Paperback Library, 1973.

Lamott, Kenneth, *Escape From Stress,* Berkley Medallion Books, 1976.

Lecker, Sidney, *The Natural Way to Control Stress,* Grosset and Dunlap, 1978.

Levinson, Harry, *Executive Stress,* Harper and Row, 1966.

Pelletier, Kenneth R., *Mind as Healer, Mind as Slayer,* Delta, 1977.

Selye, Hans, *The Stress of Life,* McGraw-Hill, 1956.

Woolfolk, Robert L. and Frank C. Richardson, *Stress, Sanity and Survival,* Monarch Press, 1978.

Yates, Jere E., *Your Own Worst Enemy,* Stephen Bosustow Productions, 1978.

—— *Managing Stress: A Businessperson's Guide,* AMACOM Publications, 1979.

Articles

Benson, Herbert, Jamie B. Kotch, Karen D. Crassweller and Martha M. Greenwood, "Historical and Clinical Considerations of the Relaxation Response," *American Scientist,* July-August 1977.

Glass, David C., "Stress Behavior Patterns and Coronary Disease," *American Scientist,* March-April 1977.

Peters, Ruanne K., and Herbert Benson, "Time Out from Tension," *Harvard Business Review,* January-February 1978.

Pines, Maya, "Psychological Hardiness," *Psychology Today,* December 1980.

Reports and Studies

Caplan, Robert D., et al. "Job Demands and Worker Health: Main Effects and Occupational Differences," U.S. Department of Health, Education and Welfare, 1975.

Editorial Research Reports: "Stress in Modern Life," 1970 Vol. II, p. 527.

Kiev, Ari and Vera Kohn, "Executive Stress," American Management Associations, 1979.

CAFFEINE CONTROVERSY

by

Marc Leepson

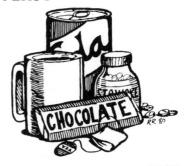

Oct. 17
1 9 8 0

Editor's Note: One reflection of the public's growing concern about the health effects of caffeine has been the introduction of 10 new cola and pepper caffeine-free soft drinks since 1980 when Royal Crown brought out the first sugar-free, caffeine-free cola, RC 100. The Food and Drug Administration's decision to remove caffeine from the group of food additives classified as "generally regarded as safe" (the GRAS list) is still pending, as is the agency's proposal that the names "cola" and "pepper" be allowed to appear on beverages that are caffeine-free *(p. 189)*.

CAFFEINE CONTROVERSY

YOU ARE running late in the morning and have time for only a cup of coffee. You drink a second cup at the mid-morning work break, and wash down lunch with a 12-ounce cola drink. For a late afternoon pick-me-up you have another cup of coffee, along with a chocolate candy bar. Before leaving for home you take two tablets of an over-the-counter headache remedy that's supposed to be more powerful than aspirin. In the evening you drink a pepper beverage at dinner. After the meal, you linger over two cups of strong tea. You drink a cup of hot chocolate before retiring for the night. In this day you have consumed about 600 milligrams of caffeine, more than the average American adult does,[1] but much less than the truly heavy coffee drinker.

Caffeine is a chemical compound found naturally in coffee beans, tea leaves, cocoa beans and kola nuts. Caffeine is added to over-the-counter and prescription drugs used as pain-relievers and stimulants. It also is added to cola drinks and to other soft drinks[2] not usually thought of as caffeine-containing beverages, such as Mountain Dew, Mello Yello and Sunkist Orange. Caffeine is a bitter-tasting, odorless drug, an alkaline in the xanthine chemical family.

Experts say caffeine is the world's most widely consumed stimulant, primarily due to the enormous popularity of coffee, tea and cola drinks. Caffeine and the other two alkaloids (theophylline and theobromine) found in these substances stimulate the central nervous system, entering all of the body's organs and tissues minutes after ingestion. Caffeine causes the heart and lungs to quicken their normal pace, the kidneys to produce more fluid and the stomach to excrete more acid. This substance also acts to clear the mind, and has a well-known property of combatting fatigue.

Recent FDA Warning to Pregnant Women

While medical science knows of these immediate effects of caffeine on the human body, the long-term consequences of heavy caffeine consumption are not known. Excessive caffeine

---

[1] According to statistics compiled by Arthur W. Burg, a biochemist at the research firm of Arthur D. Little, the average adult consumes 2.4 milligrams of caffeine a day per kilogram of body weight. That translates to about 163 milligrams for a 150-pound person. Burg derived his figures from a survey of household menus conducted by the Market Research Corp. of America. That survey included data from 4,000 households (some 12,000 individuals) during a 12-month period in 1972-73.

[2] Soft drinks generally are defined as beverages containing carbonated water, flavoring and a sweet syrup.

use has been implicated in a number of health problems, including birth defects, bladder cancer, breast disorders in women and hyperactivity in children. But thus far it has not been proven conclusively that excessive caffeine consumption causes any of these ailments in humans. In the last decade, studies have indicated that caffeine causes birth defects — including cleft palates and missing fingers and toes — in the offspring of laboratory animals fed large doses of the substance. The results of these tests prompted three consumer groups — the Center for Science in the Public Interest, the Federation of Homemakers and the Lehigh Valley Committee Against Health Fraud — to ask the U.S. Food and Drug Administration (FDA) to warn pregnant women of the possible harmful effects.

A review of caffeine conducted for the agency in 1978 recommended further study to determine long-term health implications.[3] As a result of that recommendation, the FDA and the soft drink and coffee industries began studying the possible link between heavy caffeine use and birth defects. The first phase of the agency's tests was completed in August. The results prompted FDA Commissioner Jere E. Goyan to issue a warning announcement to pregnant women Sept. 4:

> Today I am advising pregnant women to avoid caffeine-containing foods and drugs, or to use them sparingly. We know that caffeine crosses the placenta and reaches the fetus. We know that caffeine is a stimulant and has a definite drug effect. As a general rule, pregnant women should avoid all substances that have drug-like effects. So while further evidence is being gathered on the possible relationship between caffeine and birth defects, a prudent and protective mother-to-be will want to put caffeine on her list of unnecessary substances which she should avoid.

Reaction from industry and consumer groups followed a familiar pattern: Industry spokesmen said the agency went too far and consumer groups said the agency did not go far enough. The coffee and soft drink industries said the tests did not prove that caffeine causes birth defects, and thus the warning to pregnant women was premature. "The evidence is very weak," said Dr. Irwin Miller, scientific adviser to the National Coffee Association. "Dr. Goyan is counseling moderation for pregnant women, and I don't believe anybody would sanely criticize such counsel. But to single out a particular food or beverage to point to, on the basis of the kind of scientific evidence that we have today, I think is to go too far." Miller also critized the methods used in the study:

---

[3] The review, "Evaluation of the Health Aspects of Caffeine as a Food Ingredient," was prepared for FDA by the Life Sciences Research Office of the Federation of American Societies for Experimental Biology of Bethesda, Md.

Caffeine Content of Foods and Drugs

PRODUCT	CAFFEINE (mgs)
Coffee *(5 oz.)*	
Regular Brewed	
Percolated	110
Dripolator	150
Instant	66
Decaf Brewed	4.5
Instant Decaf	2
Instant or Brewed Tea *(5 oz.)*	45
Soft Drinks *(12 oz.)*	
Dr. Pepper	61
Mr. Pibb	57
Mountain Dew	49
Tab	45
Coca-Cola	42
RC Cola	36
Pepsi-Cola	35
Diet Pepsi	34
Pepsi Light	34
Cocoa *(5 oz.)*	13
Milk Chocolate *(1 oz.)*	6
Drugs *(per tablet)*	
Vivarin Tablets	200
Nodoz	100
Excedrin	65
Vanquish	33
Emperin Compound	32
Anacin	32
Dristan	16.2

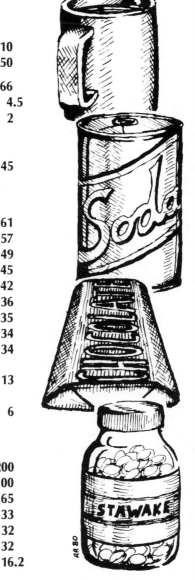

Source: Center for Science in the Public Interest

Study after study with rats has shown that when large quantities of coffee or caffeine-bearing water are given to rats in the way that the FDA did, namely by infusing it into the animal's stomach through a tube, all at once, that in large doses you get some birth defects. . . . But the doses are, first, well above what humans normally consume. But more importantly than that, the studies in which we get these effects, like the FDA study, are ones in which the material is put into the stomach by a tube all at once, not sipped slowly as humans drink coffee through the day.[4]

Dr. Howard Roberts, National Soft Drink Association vice president for science and technology, also expressed skepticism about the results of the study. He said the method of injecting caffeine directly into the rats' stomachs — called the gavage method — is not a reliable indicator of how caffeine works in the human body. "Our basic feeling was that the FDA action was not warranted," Roberts told Editorial Research Reports. Dr. Roberts' advice: "I think pregnant women should practice moderation in all aspects of their diet and physical activity — and that includes sex — and follow their doctors' advice."

The Center for Science in the Public Interest on Nov. 15, 1979, petitioned the FDA to put labels on coffee and tea packages containing caffeine to warn women about the possibility of birth defects. Michael Jacobson, a microbiologist and the center's executive director, said: "I'm very pleased that at long last FDA has come out and begun warning pregnant women to cut down on caffeine. However, I'm very disappointed that they have decided not to use the single most effective way of reaching women — that's by putting a warning notice on coffee and tea."[5]

Jacobson interprets the results of the FDA tests differently than do the coffee and soft drink industry spokesmen. "I think that it's been definitely proven that caffeine causes birth defects in animals," Jacobson said the day the warning was announced. "It has caused birth defects in mice, rats, hamsters and rabbits — four species — with missing fingers and toes showing up in several of them. . . . That's beyond a shadow of a doubt."

Agency's Experience With Saccharin Ban

The FDA's experience with caffeine typifies one of the agency's thorniest regulatory problems: deciding what action, if any, to take when scientific evidence strongly suggests, but does not prove conclusively, that a food additive causes health problems. Part of this problem can be traced to the agency's

---

[4] Appearing on the PBS-TV show, "The MacNeil/Lehrer Report," Sept. 4, 1980.
[5] Interview, Sept. 12, 1980.

experience with saccharin, the artificial sweetener. In March 1977, the FDA proposed to ban saccharin after tests by Canadian scientists showed that among laboratory rats the incidence of bladder cancer increased when the animals were fed large doses of the substance. Soon after the proposed ban was announced, Congress was deluged with complaints from angry constituents who said they needed saccharin because of illness or obesity requiring a sugar-free diet. Some members of Congress said they received more mail and phone calls on the saccharin issue than they had on any other subject in years.

In the Canadian tests, two generations of rats were fed enough of the sweetener to constitute 5 percent of their diet. Humans would have to drink about 800 12-ounce cans of diet soda a day to get an equivalent dose. That fact was stressed by those who argued that the Canadian study was meaningless for humans. They said that FDA had overreacted and should have taken into account the benefits as well as the risks of saccharin. Congress, under pressure from consumers and from diet food and drink manufacturers, overruled FDA's proposal to ban saccharin. Congress placed a moratorium on the ban in 1977, and extended the moratorium last year to June 30, 1981.

Congress, however, did not overturn an FDA ruling that saccharin-flavored products bear warning labels and that stores selling such products post warning notices. The warning label, which is found on diet soft drinks and other foods and drinks containing saccharin, reads: "Use of this product may be hazardous to your health. This product contains saccharin, which has been determined to cause cancer in laboratory animals." Under the so-called Delaney Clause,[6] a 1958 amendment to the Federal Food, Drug and Cosmetic Act of 1938, any substance found in laboratory tests to cause cancer in humans or animals must be banned — even if some putatively safe level for human food can be established.

FDA officials say that the experience with saccharin has influenced their views on regulating other food additives. "When we made the saccharin announcement [in March 1977], *The New York Times* reported that people were flooding into stores to buy it," said Richard Cooper, the FDA's former general counsel. "That is worrisome. You worry about whether the scientific case will satisfy the public and press. You can win in the scientific forum and lose in the political forum."[7]

Dr. Sanford Miller, director of FDA's Bureau of Foods, which

---

[6] Named for Rep. James J. Delaney, D-N.Y., who sponsored the amendment.
[7] Quoted in *The New York Times*, Jan. 8, 1980.

develops the agency's policy, standards and regulations on food additives, told Editorial Research Reports that the saccharin experience did not have a direct bearing on the agency's decision regarding caffeine. "No, it did not play a role in this case," Miller said. "But it has played a role in our thinking on the whole question of approaching warning labels. The experiences we had with saccharin and other warning labels we've tried very much colors our view about how to deal with susceptible segments of the population," such as pregnant women in the case of caffeine.

Questions Over the Government's Timing

Did the FDA take into account the economic aspects of caffeine? After all, the American coffee and soft drink industries are multi-billion-dollar enterprises *(see p. 193)*. "Our view on that subject is as follows," Miller said. "If we were proposing a ban — and if we do propose a ban — on the use of caffeine in colas or coffee, then I think the economic issues would play a very important role. . . . However, the fundamental decisions at least as far as this bureau is concerned will be made on the public health considerations. But . . . rarely is the data so overwhelming that other issues are not going to play a role. I would say that that would only come into play if you are moving in the direction of a ban. And that is not where we are at this point."

The caffeine study, directed by Dr. Thomas F. X. Collins, a member of the FDA's division of toxicology, was completed Aug. 1, 1980. The study examined 300 pregnant rats over an 18-month period. After the agency announced its warning to pregnant women, questions were raised about the timing of the announcement since the results of the study agreed with the findings of similar tests conducted during the last decade. Could the same warning have been issued much earlier?

"It is true that there has been a lot of animal data over the last 10 years that supports the idea that caffeine is a teratogen [causes birth defects] in animals," Miller said. "No one denies that fact — even the soft drink and the coffee people don't argue that. The argument was: Does it cause birth defects at levels which would be of concern to people? The problem has been that none of the studies were done well enough, with enough skill and care and designed properly enough to be able to answer the question unequivocally."

Miller contends that the Collins study was the first one to meet those qualifications. "Collins' study is simply the best study of its kind," he said. "It simply, unequivocally, demonstrates that indeed caffeine is a teratogen in rats at levels which are not too far different from that to which humans might be exposed.... We've gotten political pressure on the issue as a generic regulatory problem. In other words, no one has been after us because it's caffeine, but in a kind of general sense over the regulation issue of the 1980 election. I would say ... there has been no political pressure."

The FDA took other steps when it issued the warning to pregnant women. The agency (1) asked the U.S. Public Health Service to advise pregnant women about caffeine use through the service's maternal and child health projects, community health centers and other programs; (2) called on the U.S. Surgeon General to urge health professional organizations, such as the American Medical Association and the American College of Obstetricians and Gynecologists, to notify their members about the Collins study results and caffeine warning; and (3) proposed that the names "cola" and "pepper" be allowed to appear on beverages that are caffeine-free.[8] Under current regulations all beverages using those names must contain caffeine due to a "food standardization" ruling designed to insure that generically named foods contain certain ingredients.

The FDA also announced it will sponsor additional caffeine tests, due to be completed in 1981, continuing the work of the Collins study. In contrast to the gavage method used in the first study, the new tests will use the sipping method, in which caffeine is added to the rats' drinking water. The reason for the second study, Commissioner Goyan said Sept. 4, is that "scientific evidence on caffeine is inconclusive. We must seek resolution on the issues through further evaluation and research." Research projects on caffeine and birth defects also are being carried out by the International Life Sciences Institute, an industry-sponsored research organization. It is headed by Alex Malaspina, an official of the Coca-Cola Co.

Finally, the FDA announced its intention to remove caffeine from the so-called GRAS list, a group of some 400 food additives classified as "generally regarded as safe." These substances are exempt from regulation because they had long been in use when a law became effective in 1958 creating FDA's current food additive regulations.[9] The removal of caffeine from the GRAS list transfers the substance to an "interim" list. This allows manufacturers to continue to use caffeine as a food additive[10] pending the results of the FDA and industry-sponsored tests.

---

[8] The FDA itself is the agency that acts on the proposal, but it can do so only after a lengthy procedure that includes public hearings.
[9] See "Food Additives," *E.R.R.*, 1978 Vol. I, pp. 341-360.
[10] Caffeine found naturally in coffee, tea, cocoa and kola nuts is not regulated.

Popularity of Coffee and Cola

HISTORIANS do not know exactly when humans first discovered that the beans of the coffee tree could be picked, dried, hulled, ground and brewed into a beverage. It is known that Africans in what is now Ethiopia crushed dried coffee beans and mixed them with fat to eat as a food, beginning around the year 800. And it is believed that coffee probably was first grown in that area. Etymologists think that coffee derives its name either from Kaffa, a southwest Ethiopian province, or the Arabic word for the beverage, *kahwa*. According to one account: "From Ethiopia the coffee tree was taken to southern Arabia, probably by Arab slave traders or by captured slaves, and taken into cultivation some 500 years ago."[11]

Merchant companies, colonizers and missionaries took coffee seeds and seedlings throughout the world in the following centuries. Coffee drinking spread first to Persia, then to Turkey, continental Europe, the British Isles and the Americas during the 16th and 17th centuries. The first coffeehouse opened in London in 1652, and about 1689 in Boston, New York and Philadelphia. Coffee cultivation spread from Yemen in the southern Arabian Peninsula to Ceylon in 1658, Haiti and Santo Domingo in 1715, Martinique in 1723, Brazil in 1727 and elsewhere in the Caribbean, Central and South America by the mid-19th century.

Tea has been known to history much longer than coffee has. The birth of tea as a beverage has been traced in Chinese legend to 2737 B.C., and a written reference to it appeared as early as the fourth century B.C. in a Chinese dictionary. Historians believe that tea cultivation began in the province of Szechwan before spreading throughout China and, centuries later, to Japan. The Dutch are credited with introducing tea to continental Europe early in the 17th century. But it was in England where the drink enjoyed its greatest popularity in the West.

The British East India Company controlled the great spice and tea trade, and it was Parliament's attempt to extend that monopoly to the American colonies through the Tea Act of 1773 that precipitated the Boston Tea Party, foreshadowing the War of Independence. Partly as a result of that disagreement over tea, the drink never became as popular in the United States as it did in England. By 1950, Americans drank 25 times more coffee than tea, while Britons consumed five times more tea than coffee.

---

[11] Bengt A. Kihlman, *Caffeine and Chromosomes* (1977), p. 40. Kihlman is a Swedish biochemist.

Caffeine Controversy

Cocoa, unlike tea and coffee, is of New World origin. The cocoa tree, from which cocoa powder and chocolate are derived, is a native of Cental and South America. The Mayas and Aztecs used cocoa as a beverage. Christopher Columbus introduced cocoa beans to Europe in 1502, and the Europeans added vanilla and sugar to the drink. Chocolate was sold as a beverage in London in the mid-17th century, but only the rich could afford it. Though expensive, chocolate came to the British North American Colonies and its use was unimpeded by the political stigma attached to tea. Today the United States uses about 30 percent of the world's exports of raw cocoa, mostly to make eating chocolate, cocoa and cocoa butter.

Caffeine is found in three substances — guarana, maté and yoco — that are used almost exclusively in South America. Guarana, a beverage with a high caffeine content, is derived from the seeds of two plants indigenous to the Amazon Valley of Brazil. It also is eaten in solid form. Maté, also called Paraguay tea, is made from the leaves of a plant that grows wild near the Parana, Uruguay and Paraguay Rivers. A sweet drink is made of ground maté and sugar. Yoco, made from the bark of a tree that grows in southern Colombia, Ecuador and Peru, is closely related to guarana and is used as a food or a beverage.

Another caffeine-containing substance, the kola nut, is widely consumed throughout the world as a stimulant. In South America it is often chewed in solid form, especially by Indians, but kola nuts grow on evergreen trees found in South America and also in the West Indies and West Africa. Nigeria is the leading exporter of kola nuts; in North America and Europe they are used in beverages and pharmaceuticals, usually over-the-counter and prescription stimulants and pain-relievers.

Development of the Soft Drink Industry

Back in 1886, an Atlanta pharmacist named John S. Pemberton concocted a syrup containing kola nut extract, an extra dose of caffeine and coca leaf — a South American plant that has stimulating properties but not caffeine. Soon afterward the syrup was sold as a headache remedy at a number of drugstores in Atlanta under the label Coca-Cola. It was mixed first with tap water, and later with carbonated water.

Charles Howard Candler, son of the founder of the Coca-Cola Co., Asa G. Candler, wrote in an unpublished 1952 manuscript about the beverage's origins. Caffeine was used, Candler wrote, to "make it a headache remedy, starting as they did with Dr. Pemberton's Wine-Cola which had in it the stimulating Extract of Coca leaves; by eliminating the wine and increasing the sugar in the formula and adding an acid for zest, they probably got a medicine which ... had a far from pleasant

Composition of Coca-Cola

Since its inception in 1886, Coca-Cola has contained an extract of coca. This has given rise to rumors that the widely consumed drink once contained — or continues to contain — the drug cocaine, which is derived from coca leaves. An article on the subject in *The Wall Street Journal* on March 6, 1980, said it is "doubtful" that there ever was any cocaine in Coca-Cola or in any other cola drinks. Cocaine is extracted from coca leaves before they are shipped to cola makers. The cocaine is sold to pharmaceutical companies.

The fact that the exact ingredients in Coca-Cola have been a well-kept secret has fed the cocaine rumors. "The company concedes Coke contains these ingredients," *The Wall Street Journal* said: "Water, sweetener, caramel, phosphoric acid, cinnamon, vanilla, caffeine, nutmeg, lime juice, lavender, glycerin and guarana." It also contains "Merchandise No. 5: three parts coca leaves to one part cola nut." The Coca-Cola Co. lists only the following ingredients on its labels: carbonated water, sugar, caramel color, phosphoric acid, natural flavorings, caffeine.

taste. They contributed to the bitterish taste of their concoction by including in the formula some fluid extract of Kola."[12]

Coca-Cola was touted originally as a cure for exhaustion, dyspepsia, hangovers and headaches. But from its beginnings the beverage also was advertised as a delicious and refreshing treat. Both the curative and nutritive properties were illustrated in an advertisement that appeared in national magazines in the fall of 1961. The ad pictured two tired female shoppers sitting at a coffee shop table drinking Coca-Cola. The copy read: "What a Refreshing New Feeling ... what a special zing ... you get from Coke! The cold crisp taste and lively lift of Coca-Cola sends you back shopping with zest. No wonder Coke refreshes you best."

Even today the stimulation provided by the caffeine in cola and pepper drinks remains a factor in their wide popularity. "What do people expect out of a cola drink? Not only the taste, but a kick," said Sanford Miller of the FDA. "All of a sudden there is a proliferation of non-cola beverages containing caffeine — a whole bunch of citrus beverages — like Sunkist Orange Drink or Mountain Dew." The soft drink companies do not say that caffeine is added to non-cola drinks for its stimulating effects, Miller said. "They claim that it rounds out the flavor and all that kind of stuff, but the reason it's added is because it gives you a kick. The amount in the drink is enough so that if you finish one serving you're going to get a kick. It's mild, but nevertheless it is a kick."

---

[12] Quoted by Pat Watters in *Coca-Cola: An Illustrated History* (1978), p. 14.

Top Ten Soft Drinks, 1979

Drink	Percent of the U.S. Market	Drink	Percent of the U.S. Market
1. Coca-Cola*	23.9	6. Sprite	2.9
2. Pepsi-Cola*	17.9	7. Royal Crown Cola*	2.8
3. Seven Up	5.6	8. Mountain Dew*	2.7
4. Dr. Pepper*	5.5	9. Diet Pepsi*	2.5
5. Tab*	3.0	10. Diet Seven Up	1.1

*Contains caffeine
Source: *Beverage Industry* magazine, April 25, 1980

Cola drinks dominate the $13-billion-a-year American soft drink market *(see table above).* The best-selling soft drink in this country is Coca-Cola, which last year accounted for 23.9 percent of all soft drink sales, according to statistics compiled by *Beverage Industry* magazine. Pepsi-Cola followed with 17.9 percent of the market. Seven-Up (sometimes advertised as the "un-cola" to emphasize that it contains no caffeine) had 5.6 percent of the market. Dr. Pepper, which contains caffeine, followed with 5.5 percent. Sales of all Coca-Cola products last year totaled just under $5 billion. And the beverage, which *The New York Times* called "probably the one product most symbolic and symptomatic of the American way of life,"[13] today is sold in some 134 foreign countries, including China.

The National Soft Drink Association reports that soft drinks are the most popular beverages in the United States, accounting for about one-fourth of all beverages sold. Association statistics indicate that consumption of soft drinks has risen at a 7.5 percent annual rate since 1974. Analysts predict that the industry will continue to grow at an annual rate of about 3 to 4 percent in the next several years. The most recent figures show that the annual American per capita consumption of soft drinks is 382.7 12-ounce servings, making soft drinks more popular than coffee or milk.

Global Economic Importance of Coffee

Coffee, too, has economic importance. Coffee is America's largest agricultural import. It is the second biggest commodity in international trade, surpassed only by petroleum. The world's coffee-exporting nations sold some 63 million bags of coffee to other nations last year, according to the International Coffee Organization (ICO), which contends that coffee is the world's most popular drink. About one-third of the world's population drinks the beverage. ICO exporting countries sold some $11 billion worth of coffee in 1978, the last year for which complete monetary statistics are available. The United States, by far

---

[13] Dec. 20, 1978.

the leading coffee importer, bought about one-third of all coffee exports.[14]

Coffee obviously remains popular in America. However, per capita consumption has been decreasing by about 2 percent a year since 1962, when it hit a peak of 3.12 cups per day.[15] ICO statistics indicate that the average American drinks 2.02 cups of coffee a day. Almost 75 percent of the population drank coffee in 1962, compared to 56.6 percent today.

ICO began keeping statistics on decaffeinated coffee consumption three years ago. Since then the percentage of persons who drink decaffeinated coffee has risen 2.5 percent, and it accounts for 13 percent of the coffee drinkers today. Coffee industry analysts say that the number of decaffeinated coffee drinkers increased while overall coffee consumption declined basically because of improvements in the taste of de- caffeinated coffee and growing public concern about excessive caffeine consumption.

Old and New Ways of Removing Caffeine

The first decaffeination process was patented in 1907 by a German entrepreneur, Dr. Ludwig Roselius. He named the decaffeinated beverage Sanka, a word derived from the French *sans* (without) caffeine. After success in Europe, Roselius started making the beverage available in the United States but suffered a setback during World War I when, as a German, his U.S. operation was seized by the government. Though it was returned to him after the war, Roselius sold Sanka's U.S. trademark to General Foods Corp. in 1932.

The method Roselius used to decaffeinate coffee beans remains the basic process used today. The unroasted coffee beans are steamed until they are soft enough for the caffeine to be removed with a chemical solvent. The coffee beans then are processed in the usual manner: They are washed, steamed, dried, roasted and ground.

"Today, most — if not all — decaffeinated coffee manufacturers in the United States use chemical solvents to separate the caffeine," wrote Chris Lecos, a member of FDA's public affairs staff. "One of two basic methods is used: Some apply the solvent directly to the bean — the direct contact method. Others use heated water first — the water extract method

---

[14] Of the 62.85 million bags of coffee imported worldwide last year, the United States bought 21.45 million bags, about 34 percent. Brazil, the largest exporting nation, last year sold some 12 million bags, about 19 percent of the world's exports. Colombia was the second-leading exporter, followed by Ivory Coast, Indonesia and El Salvador.

[15] The drop in coffee consumption, analysts say, has been caused mainly by price increases. Coffee prices hit an all-time high in 1977 of $4.75 a pound, primarily due to a frost that severely damaged Brazil's 1975 coffee crop. Coffee prices have averaged around $3 a pound this year, but a current coffee glut could cause prices to fall by the end of the year.

American Coffee Consumption

Type	Cups Per Person Per Day				Changes
	1962	1977	1979	1980	1962-80
Regular	2.45	1.30	1.42	1.39	−1.06
Instant	0.67	0.64	0.62	0.62	−0.05
Decaf- feinated	—	0.27	0.33	0.34	—
All coffee	3.12	1.94	2.06	2.02	−1.10

Source: International Coffee Organization

— to extract the caffeine and then use the solvent to separate the caffeine from the resulting solution."[16] A third method involves using pure water instead of chemicals. One reason manufacturers are turning to the water method is that infinitesimal amounts of the decaffeinating agent wind up on the coffee beans. This has raised questions about the toxicity of the chemicals used in the process.

Today, nearly all decaffeinators use methylene chloride as the extracting agent. But until five years ago another chemical, Trichloroethylene (TCE), was used extensively. TCE use ended in July 1975 after the National Cancer Institute found that laboratory mice fed large doses of the substance developed cancer. Although FDA has not banned TCE (the agency is still testing the substance), the National Cancer Institute findings influenced decaffeinated coffee makers to stop using it.

The National Cancer Institute currently is testing methylene chloride, which, like TCE, is a chlorinated hydrocarbon. Ingestion tests on laboratory animals are scheduled to be concluded by the end of this year. In the meanwhile, the decaffeinated coffee manufacturers have been experimenting with other methods, including the use of water. The caffeine that is extracted in the decaffeination process is sold to soft drink and pharmaceutical companies. Under current FDA rules cola manufacturers are not permitted to sell decaffeinated cola beverages. But with the Sept. 4 FDA proposal to allow decaffeinated colas, industry analysts say that a number of these products will be on the market soon.[17]

There are many types of tea available today that do not contain caffeine. These include alfalfa, Irish moss, watercress, chickweed, lemon grass, hibiscus and rose hips. In addition, in the last several years tea producers have developed a process of decaffeination for tea leaves that do contain caffeine.

---

[16] Writing in *FDA Consumer*, May 1980, p. 24.
[17] The Royal Crown Cola Co. recently began marketing a new caffeine-free, sugarless cola drink called RC 100.

Other Health Implications

THE FOOD AND DRUG Administration's warning to pregnant women dealt only with the issue of caffeine and birth defects. Caffeine, though, has been linked to a number of other health problems, including bladder cancer, breast disorders in women and hyperactivity in children. As is the case with caffeine and birth defects, it has not been proven scientifically that caffeine causes these problems. The evidence accumulated thus far is what scientists call "anecdotal" — evidence that strongly hints that excessive caffeine consumption causes specific health problems but has not proven the link conclusively.

The unclear results of the scientific tests and the inability of researchers to pin down the exact cause-and-effect relationships put the FDA in a difficult regulatory position. "I keep saying we're dealing with 'beyond the frontiers,' " said Sanford Miller. "The public is asking us to do things which science isn't quite ready to do. But they want it. They want a better quality of life. And that's right. They pay the bills. Unfortunately, we don't have the means of doing it and we don't have the resources to go out and do it ourselves."

For more than a decade, scientists have been investigating whether caffeine is a cause of cancer of the bladder. A statistical association between coffee drinking and bladder cancer in New England women was reported by Philip Cole of the Harvard School of Public Health in 1971. However, Cole's findings, published that year in the British medical journal *The Lancet*, did not conclude that bladder cancer is caused by caffeine. Cole's tests found that a significant number of victims of bladder cancer were heavy caffeine users. He therefore recommended that the subject be investigated more fully.

Cole was looking into the relationship between two other factors (occupation and smoking) and bladder cancer. His discovery of the possible link between caffeine consumption and bladder cancer was a "surprise association," said Dr. Joseph Lyon, associate professor in the department of family and community medicine at the University of Utah.[18] "Cole put caffeine in as what they call a 'dummy variable.' It's one you sometimes just stick in a study to test whether people are giving you honest answers to other variables. He was rather surprised when it came out as the most significant of all the variables he had in the studies. There have been several attempts since then to verify and they have been variable. Some have found an association and some have not."

[18] Interview, Sept. 12, 1980.

One problem with these studies is the difficulty in finding people who do not drink coffee. Dr. Lyon and several University of Utah colleagues think they may have the answer in tests they currently are conducting. These tests are looking into the relationship between caffeine and bladder cancer by using some subjects who are members of the Church of Latter-day Saints (Mormons), a group whose religious teachings forbid the use of caffeine. "In this population where coffee drinking is so much different from other places in the United States, it's one of the few places we think we can get a measure of coffee drinking that might show whether it also works as a carcinogen on the bladder," said Dr. Lyon.

Breast Disease and Hyperactivity Research

For the last two years, Dr. John P. Minton of the Ohio State University College of Medicine has been studying the relationship between caffeine consumption and the development of non-cancerous fibrocystic breast disease in women. The symptoms are breast lumps and breast pain that occur about two weeks before the onset of menstruation. Minton studied 47 women who had the disease and who each drank about four cups of coffee a day.

Twenty women followed his advice to stop consuming coffee, tea, colas, chocolate and all other substances containing caffeine. Of that group 13 said that the painful breast lumps disappeared within six months. Of the 27 women who continued to consume caffeine, only one reported that the symptoms had disappeared. "Long-term followup shows continued resolution of breast symptoms and signs as long as methylxanthine [caffeine found in coffee, tea, certain soft drinks and drugs] abstinence is continued," Minton said. "The breast disease returns when methylxanthine consumption is resumed."[19]

Dr. Minton is conducting further research to try to determine what happens chemically in the body that would cause caffeine-connected breast pains. Other doctors and cancer experts say that his study does not prove that caffeine causes any of the many types of breast disorders. The prevailing medical opinion is that much more research should be completed before women with these kinds of problems should feel compelled to stop consuming caffeine.

Some researchers believe that ingesting large amounts of caffeine causes psychological problems, especially in children. Few studies have been completed, but there are some known effects of excessive caffeine consumption in children. Medical researchers say that a child consuming five cola drinks and three choco-

---

[19] Quoted in *Nutrition Action,* the monthly publication of the Center for Science in the Public Interest, August 1980, p. 4.

late bars a day is the equivalent of an adult drinking eight cups of coffee a day.

"I personally believe that there is enough evidence and logic to require that the FDA forbid the use of caffeine until industry can prove that it's completely safe to children," Michael Jacobson of the Center for Science said. "Children are heavy consumers of soft drinks. . . . Caffeine clearly causes insomnia, will cause jumpiness and fidgetiness in children. It's just not worth having that extra little nuisance in life. . . . There is evidence suggesting that caffeine will cause sleeplessness or increased motor activity in children, many of whom consume a couple of quarts of caffeinated colas a day."[20]

The Food and Drug Administration is not convinced that caffeine causes these problems in children. The agency questions the reliability of behavioral studies that indicate excessive caffeine consumption causes hyperactivity. "What we're dealing with is black magic in a sense," Sanford Miller said. "When you're dealing with behavioral issues, what [measurements] do you use? The animal behaviorist or even the human behaviorist can use things involving some kind of learning situation or he can use some kind of response to a bell. But these don't really measure behavior. . . . Theoretically, there should be an effect on developing nervous systems. But the definitive work just hasn't been done. In fact, the work that has been done and done well simply doesn't show any effect. They show effects while the kids are being exposed to the caffeine, but no long-term effect."

Dr. John Greden, associate professor of psychiatry at the University of Michigan Medical Center, has conducted research indicating that persons who consume large amounts of caffeine score high on anxiety tests. Greden also found that when heavy caffeine users stop all use of the substance, they sometimes experience intense headaches within 24 hours. "Many individuals plagued with recurrent 'tension headaches' might actually be suffering repetitive episodes of caffeine withdrawal," Greden said. "A clue would be statements from headache sufferers that combination analgesics which contain aspirin, phenacetin and caffeine are effective in relieving the pain, whereas plain aspirin is not. Other withdrawal symptoms include drowsiness, lethargy, runny nose, irritability, a disinclination to work, nervousness, depression, and even nausea."[21]

A team of psychology researchers at Centre College in Kentucky recently completed a series of tests whose results agree

[20] Interview, Sept. 12, 1980.
[21] Quoted in *World Press Review*, May 1980, p. 57, in an article adapted from the *Canadian Consumer*, published by the Consumers' Association of Canada.

Caffeine and Heart Disease

The fact that caffeine stimulates the heart muscles has led scientists to investigate the relationship, if any, between excessive caffeine consumption and diseases of the heart, including heart attacks and cardiovascular diseases.

There has been no conclusive evidence that excessive caffeine consumption causes any types of heart disease. But beginning 17 years ago, some studies have concluded that heavy coffee drinking could be a "heart risk factor;" that is, it could be a contributing cause of heart trouble. Other studies have found no link between heavy caffeine consumption and heart problems.

with Greden's findings. The researchers found that regular caffeine consumers experienced high levels of muscle tension and anxiety after abstaining from caffeine for three or more hours. The experiment involved college-student volunteers whose caffeine consumption ranged from zero to 1,140 milligrams a day. The researchers recommended that anxiety and muscle tension "be added to the list of caffeine withdrawal symptoms, which already includes headache, irritability, drowsiness and lethargy."[22] Their findings, they wrote, "demonstrate that caffeine consumption has consequences for anxiety, muscle tension and reaction time. . . . Recent abstinence from caffeine may cause increased anxiety and muscle tension reactivity in the regular user. Caffeine . . . appears to relieve the anxiety and increase reaction time. Since these effects are apparent after a relatively short abstinence, they may contribute to the maintenance of regular caffeine use."

Finally, consider the results of an experiment of sorts conducted at the Utah State Prison at Draper. Howard Richardson, the prison's food director, began serving only decaffeinated coffee in June 1979. Some inmates reportedly were drinking as many as 20 cups of coffee a day. What's happened since decaffeinated coffee was substituted? "In the dining room there's generally a lot of hollering and yelling and you have a lot of knifing and stuff like that," Richardson said. "And I just don't think we have that many anymore."[23] As is the case with most of the studies dealing with caffeine and health problems, the Utah State Prison results are anecdotal and do not prove that caffeine causes violent behavior among prisoners. But all of the anecdotal evidence, at the very least, raises troubling questions about a substance that most people ingest nearly every day of their lives.

---

[22] Writing in *Science*, Sept. 26, 1980, p. 1548.
[23] Telephone interview, Oct. 2, 1980.

Selected Bibliography

Books

Brewster, Letitia and Michael F. Jacobson, *The Changing American Diet*, Center for Science in the Public Interest, 1978.
Dietz, Lawrence, *Soda Pop*, Simon & Schuster, 1973.
Forster, Robert and Orest Ranum, eds., *Food and Drink in History*, Johns Hopkins University Press, 1979.
Hess, John L. and Karen Hess, *The Taste of America*, Penguin, 1977.
Kihlman, Bengt A., *Caffeine and Chromosomes*, Elsevier Scientific, 1977.
Mortimer, William Golden, *History of Coca*, J. H. Vail, 1901.
Root, Waverly and Richard de Rochemont, *Eating in America*, Morrow, 1976.
Scott, J. M., *The Tea Story*, Heinemann, 1964.
Watters, Pat, *Coca-Cola: An Illustrated History*, Doubleday, 1978.
Wellman, F. L., *Coffee: Botany, Cultivation and Utilization*, Leonard Hill, 1961.

Articles

"Coffee," *The Courier*, January-February 1980.
FDA Consumer, selected issues.
Grossier, Daniel S., "A Study of Caffeine in Tea," *The American Journal of Clinical Nutrition*, October 1978.
"Instant Coffees," *Consumer Reports*, October 1979.
Jones, Chris and Gary Benson, "The Mormons: Healthy in Body and Soul," *The Saturday Evening Post*, May-June 1980.
National Coffee Association, *News Letter*, selected issues.
Nutrition Action, selected issues.
Tea & Coffee Trade Journal, selected issues.
White, Brent C., *et al.*, "Anxiety and Muscle Tension as Consequence of Caffeine Withdrawal," *Science*, Sept. 26, 1980.

Reports and Studies

Coffee Information Institute, "Safety of Caffeine-Containing Beverages," Nov. 27, 1978.
Editorial Research Reports: "Food Additives," 1978 Vol. I, p. 343.
International Coffee Organization: "The Story of Coffee," 1979; "Coffee: The World Cup," May 1979; "Summary of National Coffee Drinking Survey," winter 1980.
National Coffee Association, "Caffeine and Birth Defects: Scientific Update," June 27, 1980.
U.S. Food and Drug Administration, "Report on Caffeine," September 1980.

INDEX